Foreign Remedies: What the Experience of Other Nations Can Tell Us about Next Steps in Reforming U.S. Health Care

David A. Rochefort and Kevin P. Donnelly

W0018399

The Patient Protection and Affordable Care Act marked a watershed in U.S. health policy, but controversy over its passage rages on, and much uncertainty surrounds the law's transformation from blueprint into operational program. How can the experience of other nations help us to reconcile the competing goals of universal coverage, cost control, and high-quality care? Following an analysis of the 2010 statute, this book surveys developments in different parts of the globe to identify important lessons in health politics, policy design, and program implementation. A concluding chapter examines the issue of resistance to foreign remedies within the process of U.S. health reform.

David A. Rochefort is Arts and Sciences Distinguished Professor of Political Science at Northeastern University. His previous books include *From Poorhouses to Homelessness: Policy Analysis and Mental Health Care* (1997, 2nd ed.) and, coeditor with Robert B. Hackey, *The New Politics of State Health Policy* (2001), among other works. He has also served as a consultant to government agencies in Massachusetts, Rhode Island, New Jersey, and at the federal level.

Kevin P. Donnelly received his Ph.D. from Northeastern University in 2009 focusing on health policy and political language. He is Assistant Professor of Political Science and Public Administration at Bridgewater State University. His publications have appeared in *Harvard Health Policy Review* and *Medicine and Health Rhode Island*.

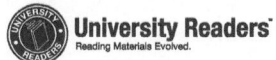 **THE SOCIAL ISSUES COLLECTION**™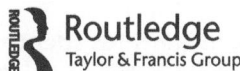

Framing 21st Century Social Issues

The goal of this new, unique Series is to offer readable, teachable "thinking frames" on today's social problems and social issues by leading scholars. These are available for view on http://routledge.customgateway.com/routledge-social-issues.html.

For instructors teaching a wide range of courses in the social sciences, the Routledge *Social Issues Collection* now offers the best of both worlds: originally written short texts that provide "overviews" to important social issues *as well as* teachable excerpts from larger works previously published by Routledge and other presses.

As an instructor, click to the website to view the library and decide how to build your custom anthology and which thinking frames to assign. Students can choose to receive the assigned materials in print and/or electronic formats at an affordable price.

Available

Body Problems
Running and Living Long in a Fast-Food Society
Ben Agger

Sex, Drugs, and Death
Addressing Youth Problems in American Society
Tammy Anderson

The Stupidity Epidemic
Worrying About Students, Schools, and America's Future
Joel Best

Empire Versus Democracy
The Triumph of Corporate and Military Power
Carl Boggs

Contentious Identities
Ethnic, Religious, and Nationalist Conflicts in Today's World
Daniel Chirot

The Future of Higher Education
Dan Clawson and Max Page

Waste and Consumption
Capitalism, the Environment, and the Life of Things
Simonetta Falasca-Zamponi

Rapid Climate Change
Causes, Consequences, and Solutions
Scott G. McNall

The Problem of Emotions in Societies
Jonathan H. Turner

Outsourcing the Womb
Race, Class, and Gestational Surrogacy in a Global Market
France Winddance Twine

Changing Times for Black Professionals
Adia Harvey Wingfield

Why Nations Go to War
A Sociology of Military Conflict
Mark P. Worrell

How Ethical Systems Change:
Eugenics, the Final Solution, Bioethics
Sheldon Ekland-Olson and Julie Beicken

How Ethical Systems Change:
Abortion and Neonatal Care
Sheldon Ekland-Olson and Elyshia Aseltine

How Ethical Systems Change:
Tolerable Suffering and Assisted
Dying
Sheldon Ekland-Olson and Elyshia Aseltine

How Ethical Systems Change:
Lynching and Capital Punishment
Sheldon Ekland-Olson and Danielle Dirks

DIY: The Search for Control and
Self-Reliance in the 21st Century
Kevin Wehr

Nuclear Family Values, Extended
Family Lives: The Power of Race,
Class, and Gender
Natalia Sarkisian and Naomi Gerstel

Disposable Youth, Racialized
Memories, and the Culture of Cruelty
Henry Giroux

Due Process Denied: Detentions and
Deportations in the United States
Tanya Golash-Boza

Oversharing: Presentation of Self
in the Internet Age
Ben Agger

Foreign Remedies: What the
Experience of Other Nations Can Tell
Us about Next Steps in Reforming
U.S. Health Care
David A. Rochefort and Kevin P. Donnelly

Forthcoming

Future Ethics
Charles Lemert and Sam Han

Sociology of Mindfulness
Jodi O'Brien

It's the Economy, Stupid
Stanley Aronowitz

HIV/AIDS: A Global Social Problem
Carrie Foote

Google Bombs, Astroturf, and
Cloaked Sites
Jessie Daniels

Girls with Guns
France Winddance Twine

Torture and Rights
Lisa Hajjar

Are We Coddling Prisoners?
Benjamin Fleury-Steiner

Sociology of Terror, Terrorism,
and Terrorists
Mark Worrell

Foreign Remedies

What the Experience of Other Nations Can Tell Us about Next Steps in Reforming U.S. Health Care

David A. Rochefort

Northeastern University

Kevin P. Donnelly

Bridgewater State University

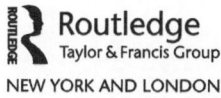

Routledge
Taylor & Francis Group

NEW YORK AND LONDON

First published 2012
by Routledge
711 Third Avenue, New York, NY 10017

Simultaneously published in the UK
by Routledge
2 Park Square, Milton Park, Abingdon, Oxon OX14 4RN

Routledge is an imprint of the Taylor & Francis Group, an informa business

Library of Congress Cataloging in Publication Data
Rochefort, David A.
    Foreign remedies : what the experience of other nations can tell us about next steps in reforming U.S. health care / David A. Rochefort, Kevin P. Donnelly.
    p. cm. — (Framing 21st century social issues)
    1. Health care reform. 2. Health care reform—United States. 3. United States. Patient Protection and Affordable Care Act. I. Donnelly, Kevin P. II. Title.
    RA395.A3R624 2012
    362.1'0425—dc23
    2011039550

ISBN13: 978-0-415-51796-6 (pbk)
ISBN13: 978-0-203-12359-1 (ebk)

Typeset in Garamond and Gill Sans
by EvS Communication Networx, Inc.

University Readers (www.universityreaders.com): Since 1992, University Readers has been a leading custom publishing service, providing reasonably priced, copyright-cleared, course packs, custom textbooks, and custom publishing services in print and digital formats to thousands of professors nationwide. The Routledge Custom Gateway provides easy access to thousands of readings from hundreds of books and articles via an online library. The partnership of University Readers and Routledge brings custom publishing expertise and deep academic content together to help professors create perfect course materials that are affordable for students.

Contents

Series Foreword

The world in the early 21st century is beset with problems—a troubled economy, global warming, oil spills, religious and national conflict, poverty, HIV, health problems associated with sedentary lifestyles. Virtually no nation is exempt, and everyone, even in affluent countries, feels the impact of these global issues.

Since its inception in the 19th century, sociology has been the academic discipline dedicated to analyzing social problems. It is still so today. Sociologists offer not only diagnoses; they glimpse solutions, which they then offer to policy makers and citizens who work for a better world. Sociology played a major role in the civil rights movement during the 1960s in helping us to understand racial inequalities and prejudice, and it can play a major role today as we grapple with old and new issues.

This series builds on the giants of sociology, such as Weber, Durkheim, Marx, Parsons, Mills. It uses their frames, and newer ones, to focus on particular issues of contemporary concern. These books are about the nuts and bolts of social problems, but they are equally about the frames through which we analyze these problems. It is clear by now that there is no single correct way to view the world, but only paradigms, models, which function as lenses through which we peer. For example, in analyzing oil spills and environmental pollution, we can use a frame that views such outcomes as unfortunate results of a reasonable effort to harvest fossil fuels. "Drill, baby, drill" sometimes involves certain costs as pipelines rupture and oil spews forth. Or we could analyze these environmental crises as inevitable outcomes of our effort to dominate nature in the interest of profit. The first frame would solve oil spills with better environmental protection measures and clean-ups, while the second frame would attempt to prevent them altogether, perhaps shifting away from the use of petroleum and natural gas and toward alternative energies that are "green."

These books introduce various frames such as these for viewing social problems. They also highlight debates between social scientists who frame problems differently. The books suggest solutions, on both the macro and micro levels. That is, they suggest what new policies might entail, and they also identify ways in which people, from the ground level, can work toward a better world, changing themselves and their lives and families and providing models of change for others.

Readers do not need an extensive background in academic sociology to benefit from these books. Each book is student-friendly in that we provide glossaries of terms for the uninitiated that are keyed to bolded terms in the text. Each chapter ends with questions for further thought and discussion. The level of each book is accessible to undergraduate students, even as these books offer sophisticated and innovative analyses.

American health care is on the lips of nearly every politician. The Patient Protection and Affordable Care Act marked a watershed in U.S. health policy, but controversy over its passage rages on, and much uncertainty surrounds the law's transformation from blueprint into operational program. How can the experience of other nations help us to reconcile the competing goals of universal coverage, cost control, and high-quality care? Following an analysis of the 2010 statute, David Rochefort and Kevin Donnelly address developments in different parts of the globe to identify important lessons in health politics, policy design, and program implementation. A concluding chapter examines the issue of resistance to foreign remedies within the process of U.S. health reform.

Preface

In early September of 2011, when Republican presidential hopefuls convened for debate at the Ronald Reagan library in Simi Valley, California, the future of Social Security sparked a lively exchange. Talk of measured reform competed with calls for abandonment of the program, providing revealing insight into the ideological leanings of politicians on the stage. Herman Cain, former CEO of Godfather's Pizza, who is also a talk radio host and Baptist minister, weighed in with these words:

> I happen to believe that, yes, Social Security, it needs fixing, not continuing to talk about it. I believe in the Chilean model, where you give a personal retirement account option so we can move this society from an entitlement society to an empowerment society ... Give them [workers] a choice with an account with their name on it, and over time we would eliminate the current broken system that we have. That is a solution to the problem. Rather than continuing to talk about how broken it is, let's just fix it using the Chilean model.
>
> (*New York Times* 2011)

For someone aiming to move from the shadows into the main pack of contenders for his party's nomination, it was a curious position for Cain to stake out, or at least to stake out in these rhetorical terms. The truth is that mainstream American political leaders rarely advocate for change by recommending the United States copy policies from other countries.

This book is about health care, not Social Security, and in no realm has American resistance to foreign policies and philosophies become more evident over time. Economically developed nations have many problems in common in the delivery, financing, and management of health services. They also confront similar disease patterns and technology advancements, with all the mixed blessings that come with the latter. Yet this shared experience and the interventions it has inspired have not influenced the formulation of U.S. health policy to a great extent. Despite urging from a number of experts, officials have typically neglected—indeed, they have often openly rejected—

the lessons of comparative policy analysis in favor of uniquely American approaches to the task of health reform.

A dramatic breakthrough in U.S. health policy occurred with passage of the Affordable Care Act in 2010, a complex piece of legislation aimed at moderating, but not eliminating, problems of insurance coverage while attempting to slow the upward spiral of health care costs. What strengths and weaknesses does the Affordable Care Act possess? What political, design, and organizational problems are likely to arise as the law enters an uncertain period of gradual implementation? How can wisdom gained from the successes and failures of health systems elsewhere around the world be utilized in coping with expected challenges? These are the principal questions addressed by this book. We also explore the process of public policy learning and, in particular, the reasons why Americans have found it so difficult to benefit from a cross-national perspective on health care issues. Whatever twists and turns lie ahead in the unfolding struggle over U.S. health reform—and no one can make exact predictions in this current turbulent political environment—our discussion highlights the enduring concerns, obstacles, and opportunities that define health care as an issue in contemporary society. Undergraduate students make up the primary audience of the *Framing 21st Century Social Issues* series to which this volume belongs, but our work is for anyone seeking a broad introduction to comparative health policy studies, written to be at once pointed and to the point.

Acknowledgements

A number of debts have been incurred in the writing of this book, and we wish to express our gratitude to key individuals here. Our thanks go, first, to Ben Agger, academic editor of the *Framing 21st Century Social Issues* series, for his invitation to write this book and to have it join the growing list of engaging social science titles he is shepherding into publication. David Mechanic, René Dubos University Professor of Behavioral Sciences and Director of the Institute for Health, Health Care Policy, and Aging Research at Rutgers University, was responsible for putting us together with Ben, and he also kindly agreed to read a draft of this work. Others who generously paused their busy schedules to comment on our manuscript included Michael S. Dukakis, Distinguished Professor of Political Science, Northeastern University, and Paul Block, Director, Psychological Centers, Providence, Rhode Island. We appreciate the encouragement given to us by these good colleagues and friends, who all helped improve this book as a final product and, of course, bear no responsibility for its limitations. Matthew Cournoyer, an outstanding undergraduate student at Northeastern University, helped enormously in the early phase of gathering research materials for this project. Leah Babb-Rosenfeld and Sarah Stone, editorial and production staff members at Routledge, handled our manuscript with skill and efficiency. Finally, we dedicate this book to our families, who patiently put up with our absences, distractions, and frustrations as we labored to whip into shape a large and ungainly topic that we believe is critical to understanding the role of government in our lives.

1: From National to Global Awareness in Health Policy Analysis

The United States has the best health care in the world. It is a claim heard often enough these days.

After President Obama launched his reform initiative in early 2009, Republican Senator Richard Shelby of Alabama labeled it the first step in "destroying the best health care system the world has ever known" (Fox News 2009). Governor Bob McDonnell echoed this point when delivering the official Republican response to the 2010 State of the Union speech: "All Americans agree, we need a health care system that is affordable, accessible, and high quality. But most Americans do not want to turn over the best medical care system in the world to the federal government" (ABC News 2010).

Just one month earlier, conservative radio host Rush Limbaugh had entered a hospital in Honolulu after developing chest pains while on Christmas holiday. Grateful for the excellent care he received, Limbaugh turned the episode into a political lesson: "I have been treated to the best healthcare the world has to offer, and that is right here in the United States of America" (Kutch 2010). Critics, however, were quick to point out a certain irony. With Hawaii's unionized hospital staffing and mandatory health insurance for those working more than 20 hours a week, Limbaugh arguably had reaped the benefits of "one of the most progressive" state health care systems in the country.

Although President Obama and his supporters ultimately won the fight for their health bill, it was Republicans who dominated House and Senate elections the following November. Reveling in victory, incoming Speaker of the House John Boehner lashed out against the Democratic legislative accomplishment in familiar terms: "[T]he healthcare bill that was enacted by the current Congress will kill jobs in America, ruin the best healthcare system in the world, and bankrupt our country" (Lawder 2010).

Many members of the public apparently share this belief in the unrivalled advantages of U.S. health care. In 2008, a national cross section of adults was asked the following question:

Some people say that the United States has the best health care system in the world. Others say that the health care systems of some other countries are better than the U.S. How about you? Do you think that in general the U.S. has the best health care system or are there other countries with better health care systems?

Results showed 45 percent thought the United States has the best system, while 39 percent believed other countries have better systems (remaining respondents either didn't know or refused to answer). Did respondents possess any factual knowledge about health care in other countries? Were they responding to this item based on personal experience with American medicine or a perception of the U.S. system in general, neither or both? Without answers to such questions, opinion findings like these defy easy interpretation. Still, it is striking how sharply divided those surveyed were. Nearly 70 percent of Republicans claimed the United States has the best health care, but only 32 percent of Democrats. Pollster Robert Blendon commented on the implications: "The health care debate ... involves starkly different views of the U.S. health care system. One party sees it as lagging [behind] other countries across a broad range of problem areas while the other party sees the system as the best in the world with a more limited range of problems" (Harvard School of Public Health 2008).

Now consider this same issue of the relative standing of U.S. health care as addressed by health policy analysts.

In 2000, the World Health Organization measured health system performance across 191 member states using five indicators: overall population health, **health disparities** between different population groups, health system responsiveness, service to people of varying economic status, and the distribution of health system costs (WHO 2000). Based on this approach, the United States ranked a poor 37th.

More recently, in 2009, the Robert Wood Johnson Foundation and the Urban Institute collaborated on a cross-national study of **health care quality**. Again, after considering multiple definitions and indicators, the authors concluded: "[T]here is no hard evidence that identifies particular areas in which U.S. health care quality is truly exceptional." And they challenged "the argument that reform of the U.S. health system stands to endanger 'the best health care quality in the world'" (Docteur and Berenson 2009: 9–10).

Prominent among other research groups investigating this subject, the Commonwealth Fund produced a series of four reports on health care performance internationally between 2004 and 2010 (Davis, Schoen, and Stremikis 2010). The latest study matches the U.S. against six other industrialized nations—Australia, Canada, Germany, The Netherlands, New Zealand, and the United Kingdom—and makes use of surveys collecting patient and physician data. By far the most expensive system, the U.S. ranked last overall within this comparison group, and no better than fourth place for any of the selected quality, access, efficiency, equity, and "healthy lives" measures.

To the question "Mirror, Mirror on the Wall, Who's the Fairest of them All?" these researchers gave a blunt reply: the U.S. rarely "outperforms" other economically developed Western nations.

Comparative ratings such as these are far from above criticism on methodological grounds (Whitman 2008; Bialik 2009). One thorny difficulty is producing an overall assessment for a country like the United States that possesses abundant resources, highly skilled professionals, and excellent medical facilities while roughly 50 million people have lacked health insurance. The WHO study has been taken to task for failing to control for health outcomes reflecting differences in the make-up and lifestyles of different populations. Recent analysis of national longevity differences indicates the powerful significance of smoking and obesity as particular factors within the United States (Crimmins, Preston, and Cohen 2011). Some health policy specialists complain, further, about competitive frameworks that pit nations against each other as if in "a sports tournament" (Marmor, Freeman, and Okma 2008). Nonetheless, when all is said and done, it is difficult to set aside consistent empirical findings identifying deficiencies of U.S. health care as a *system* of services and protections.

Here, then, a contradiction. On one side, the audacious mantra of "We're Number 1!" On the other, the well-documented problems of U.S. health care. How can we reconcile the two?

First, the former perspective has strong political undertones. It is as dogmatic in its way as the alternative extreme would be that there is little right with U.S. health care. This conclusion is consistent with the line-up of commentators extolling the present system's virtues, as well as by the partisan breakdown of survey respondents who agree with them. An indignant claim of American superiority has become rhetorical short-hand for a certain agenda in contemporary health policy making, one promising no disruptive changes in American medicine that might be associated with expanded government powers and responsibilities. It is a rallying cry many individuals and groups find appealing today, not just the professional, economic, and institutional interests vested in the status quo.

Second, if a certain superiority complex about U.S. health care may be said to exist, it also reflects values deeply resonant within American history, society, and culture. The assertion of national pre-eminence in any domain is inevitably, in part, an expression of heartfelt patriotism. More than this, it gives voice to the sense of "exceptionalism" long held by Americans in regard to "their uniqueness, their differences from the rest of the world, the vitality of their democracy, the growth potential of their economy" (Lipset 1996: 17). Such a view blends easily with an **isolationism** in which homegrown ideas and practices seem preferable almost by definition. Yet, paradoxically, this claim that "U.S. health care is best" redirects our attention abroad by making the perceived performance of others a benchmark when appraising our own situation. Put simply, to enter the realm of good-better-best is to concede the relevance of national comparisons in discussing the intricacies of health care, including public policy's role in shaping a system's organization and outcomes.

Although the United States resists flattery-through-imitation in the overt borrowing of foreign health policy ideas, a significant history of curiosity about international developments lies outside the official mainstream. Germany was a model for labor reformers who proposed compulsory health insurance legislation in many state capitols during the Progressive era (Lubove 1968). American observers showed persistent interest in British health insurance throughout the last century with a focus on two landmark laws, the National Insurance Act of 1911 and the National Health Service Act of 1946 (Land 1982). Pro-market reforms that began under Prime Minister Thatcher in the 1990s, a policy undertaken with American inspiration and consultation, have continued to capture notice for the British health system into the 21st century. After adopting a program of universal coverage built on **federalism** principles in the 1970s, Canada also became a primary object of attention for **national health insurance** advocates ranging from Senator Edward Kennedy, to Physicians for a National Health Program, to the filmmaker Michael Moore (Rochefort and Donnelly 2008).

The scholarly study often acknowledged for attracting broad interest to the field of comparative health policy is *A Healthy State*, first published by Victor and Ruth Sidel in 1977. Although previous works by academics and government researchers had delved into this topic, none succeeded so well in putting the U.S. health care "crisis" into international context for a large audience of specialists, students, and interested general readers. For Sidel and Sidel (1983), a physician and a social worker, "it is often the view from outside one's society that is most enlightening" (p. xviii). Seeking "to clarify and propose remedies for problems within the United States," they chose to concentrate on four other countries: Sweden, Great Britain, the Soviet Union, and the People's Republic of China. While big differences in financing, medical practice, institutional structure, population, and politics distinguished members of this group one from the other, all had made a commitment to **health care reform** "in a highly planned and organized way" (p. xx). And it was results of these efforts that contained potentially valuable lessons for the United States in facing its own health policy dilemmas.

In the aftermath of *A Healthy State* came a rising flood of writing—journal articles, scholarly monographs, popular books, newspaper features, and more—that set an ambitious global agenda in health policy analysis. Today this cumulative body of work assumes impressive proportions and makes possible a volume of synthesis such as our own. More than just a series of snapshots of foreign health systems unfamiliar to most Americans, a sophisticated logic of inquiry has been established through the labors of an entire generation of health policy "comparativists" (see, e.g., Stone 1981; Morone 1990; White 1995; Marmor, Freeman, and Okma 2009; Blank and Burau 2010). Essential tenets of this approach may be outlined as follows:

- Health systems are the product of socioeconomic and political conditions that are, to some extent, distinctive in each country. Simply transplanting systems from one country to another is not a realistic possibility. Instead, comparative analysis must focus on identifying those policies, principles, and practices having reasonable chance of adaptation beyond their original setting.
- An understanding of the health sector's dynamic character—its driving forces, conflicting interests, most intransigent challenges, and future directions—can be improved by noting how national systems both converge and diverge in their dominant tendencies.
- Information about health care in other countries has often been incorporated within domestic political debate for the purpose of conjuring up worst-case scenarios about where new reform proposals might lead. For this reason, the subject is rife with distortion, and myth busting has emerged as an important objective of comparative health policy analysis.
- Cultural factors shaping the organization of national health systems also shape their description. Use of similar terms to mean different things, idiosyncratic methods of data collection, and varying performance standards all must be reckoned with in any meaningful accounting of how different health systems operate.
- Not just other nations' successes, but their mistakes as well, can be valuable in learning lessons from abroad. In fact, one optimistic perspective on the U.S. position as laggard in the international movement for comprehensive coverage and cost control is that we have gained the advantage of benefiting from the missteps of other nations that boldly seized the lead in tackling this conundrum (Rodwin 1987).

With these observations in mind, as guidance and as warning, this book provides a concise review of health system developments in different parts of the globe. Our interest lies particularly with those policies, programs, and administrative practices that might usefully inform next steps as the United States seeks to consolidate and build upon recently enacted reforms. The intention is less to provide definitive answers, however, than to sharpen key options meriting debate within an unfolding process.

Contrary to the typical case-study approach in comparative analysis, a slim volume like this cannot examine even a small group of national health systems in depth. We have chosen another way to get our information across. After an opening chapter that categorizes main features of U.S. health care from an international perspective and explains the 2010 health reform law, the core presentation is structured around broad themes—societal impacts on medicine and health, the politics of health policy making, health policy design, and program implementation and management—while incorporating myriad examples from the foreign experience where these fit best. The "usual suspects" in comparative analysis—Canada, England, France, Germany, and other West European nations—come up repeatedly in this book. Yet readers will also learn something about Australia, Japan, Israel, Taiwan, and other nations that usually receive slight mention when considering the future path of U.S. health care. Issues of public policy remain our focus throughout, but the orientation is interdisciplinary, drawing on sources and perspectives from political science, sociology, history, public health, economics, public administration, and other fields.

The United States stands at a crucial juncture in health policy development. The most significant piece of reform legislation in half a century has just been passed, yet it roiled the political waters rather than calming them and organized opposition rages unabated. Moreover, not even staunchest supporters of this new law can be confident about how its complex provisions will work when put into operation, particularly given the large implementing role to be played by 50 states. How poorly or well critical tasks are handled—cost containment, resource allocation, bureaucratic management, public–private coordination, consumer protection—could easily mean the difference between success and failure. In short, at a time when creative ideas continue to be badly needed in U.S. health policy, **xenophobia** could well prove the most crippling disease of them all. Our final chapter returns to this issue of resistance toward learning foreign remedies for U.S. health care problems.

DISCUSSION QUESTIONS

1. To what extent do you think Americans' understanding of their health system has become distorted by the rhetorical spin of political leaders and special interests?
2. Do you think it is meaningful to attempt to rank different national health systems?
3. What criteria are relevant in deciding which foreign health systems should be of most interest to an American audience?

II: U.S. Health Care in Comparative Perspective

❦

Every book takes readers on a journey, this book perhaps more so than most. First, this is a travel book of sorts that covers a great deal of geography in examining health care around the globe, from the United States to elsewhere in North America, from North America to Europe, Asia, and the "down under" island continent of Australia. Second, by exploring the political, social, economic, and organizational bases of diverse health systems, this book is an intellectual trek through the ideas, interests, and operational realities of health policy making. Third, this book takes tentative steps into the unknown territory of the future, viewing the current status of U.S. health reform as a crossroads from which various paths forward are possible.

Lest this journey begin in confusion, a clear point of departure is necessary. This chapter puts the United States into comparative perspective by considering scholarly approaches for classifying national health care systems. This discussion is valuable not only as conceptual orientation, but also as backdrop for a close-up view of health care in 21st-century America. The question before us then: Where are we now?

Classifying National Health Systems

The first attempts to compare health care in different countries based on funding, coverage, and service-delivery criteria were made more than 50 years ago (Anderson 1963; Roemer 1960). Adding to this effort, in 1973 a medical sociologist at Boston University named Mark Field (1973) set for himself the ambitious task of describing the health systems of modern society. His framework included four "ideal types":

A *pluralistic health system* functions in the absence of a unified structural plan. It consists of a variety of health facilities and services exhibiting different organizational forms and operating under private and public ownership. Doctors in a pluralistic system are privately employed and maintain a high degree of professional autonomy.

A *health insurance system* also tends to be highly pluralistic organizationally with a large amount of physician independence. However, most financial payments are made by private insurers, government, and other agencies. Although the role played by third-party payers gives a basis for undertaking external supervision of the delivery of health care, a tradition of self-regulation by providers and institutions, as well as diffuse payer involvement, may block this potential from becoming reality.

A *health service system* features national ownership of most health care facilities, and physicians are paid from the public treasury. The latter, particularly those in community practice as opposed to salaried hospital positions, view themselves as private providers, enjoying the same autonomy as physicians in pluralist and health insurance systems.

A *socialized health system* is one in which the state owns and manages all facilities. Doctors and other health personnel are typically state employees, whose professional work may be subject to direct assignment and management by public authorities.

Applying his ideal types to national systems around the world, Field came up with the following pairings: pluralistic—United States; health insurance—the health systems of Western Europe and Japan; health service—Great Britain; and socialized—the Soviet Union and Eastern European nations.

Field recognized the provisional nature of his schema, which he called merely a "stab" at dealing with "formidable, theoretical, and empirical problems" (p. 773). Nonetheless, this was a milestone in clarifying the universe of health care delivery. Not only did Field's approach underscore major similarities and differences among contemporary national health systems, it also cited important implications for the "locus of control" in decision making, resource distribution, and program development.

The Organisation for Economic Co-operation and Development (OECD) outlined three basic health care systems in the late 1980s (OECD 1987). First, the *national health service* model features universal health coverage funded through general taxation. Second, the *social insurance* model refers to a system in which health care coverage is also universal, but funded and delivered primarily by private entities. Third, the *private insurance* system centers on purchase of coverage by individuals and employers, and there is private ownership of health service delivery. The United States clearly fell into this last category, a reflection of the continued dominance of insurance coverage acquired as a benefit from one's place of work.

Although widely influential, the OECD approach did little more than portray existing arrangements in a limited sample of nations (Burau and Blank 2006). Even in its updated form—the latest tripartite classification includes "public integrated," "public contract," and "private insurance-provider" models—it cannot easily be applied to all countries (OECD 2004). Consider the nations of South Korea and Taiwan. Health reforms in these countries in the 1990s yielded a high degree of government management, on the one hand, and private control of organizational resources, on the other. Taiwan is a very interesting case because its system was deliberately constructed through a process devoted to learning from the most successful features of health care provision in other industrialized countries (Reid 2009). While bearing similarity to Canada's single-payer model, or the American Medicare program, the model is distinctive from a regulatory standpoint, leading some analysts to call for more discrimination among National Health Insurance programs according to the character and values of state intervention (Lee et al. 2008).

One well-conceived attempt to go beyond description to theoretical explanation in system classification comes from Michael Moran (2000), Professor of Government at the University of Manchester. By focusing on the "systems of politics" governing consumption, provision, and technology, Moran links health care to larger welfare state issues but without simply equating the two topics.

Moran's **typology** consists of four "families." In an *entrenched command and control* state, such as the United Kingdom, the government dominates consumption and provision of health care, but plays a small role in production of medical technology. In a *corporatist* state, like Germany, "public law bodies," not the government, dominate the governance of health care, limiting direct state control. *Insecure command and control* states, represented by the Mediterranean nations of Portugal, Spain, Italy, and Greece, possess the apparatus of a *command and control* state, but with little success, in practice, displacing private interests. And the United States belongs to the final category of a *supply state*, in which vagaries of private insurance limit public access to health services, while providers and creators of medical technology operate outside government control. For Moran, the U.S. illustrates why it can be misleading to view health systems simply in terms of greater or lesser market control: "America's historical distinctiveness lay in the domination of *suppliers*, not in the domination of the market; and the American state was a dominant force in creating a supplier-dominated health economy" (Moran 2000: 155).

Julian Le Grand is an academic economist who also served as senior policy advisor to British Prime Minister Tony Blair. His approach to health policy analysis considers the means through which public ends can be pursued (Le Grand 2007). The first method Le Grand identifies is *trust*. Here government sets the overall budget for an activity while public managers are "trusted" to use resources as they see fit. Another approach establishes *targets*. Under this system, professional and organizational rewards are tied to meeting defined objectives. A third method is *voice*, which relies on users of a service to communicate satisfaction or dissatisfaction to providers in order to prompt optimization. Last, there is *choice and competition*, a context giving users leverage to choose among competing providers. Le Grand characterizes the U.S. as the nation with the most competitive health care. As a supporter of market structuring attempts within Britain's National Health Service, he finds favor with government's circumscribed role in U.S. health care, which may seem ironic given how frequently others criticize this same trait. Le Grand does, however, emphasize the choice-and-competition model can only succeed under proper regulatory conditions, many of which are absent or poorly developed in the American context.

Other typologies exist, but this abbreviated listing suffices to suggest the wide range of health system configurations across nations and how it can be depicted. No matter the vantage point, one fact is plain: the United States stands as one of the countries with the most limited government presence in the health sector, a situation leaving pivotal matters of access, service delivery, and resource allocation in private hands. The record is strong on entrepreneurialism, weak on citizenship rights and comprehensiveness.

All classifying attempts risk the pitfall that critical details will be sacrificed to over-generalization (Freeman and Frisina 2010). Although a nation may be dominated by a given health model, it does not mean others are not also present. Mixed approaches often exist in health finance, service organization, and administration, along with variation "across time and space within a single country" (Blank and Burau 2010: 15–17). Nor are the issues facing specific health sectors—acute care vs. long-term care vs. mental health vs. public health—well handled by summary categories (Mechanic and Rochefort 1996). Classification is an inherently fluid, always unfinished, task. This much is evident in the sheer proliferation of health system typologies, not to mention the habit of analysts revisiting their own frameworks to update and refine them.

The solution is not to abandon classification, but rather to combine it with appreciation of idiosyncrasies in the way national systems take form and function. The next section explores these particulars in the American setting.

A Spotlight on U.S. Health Care

Political scientist Michael Reagan (1999) has called health care in the United States an "accidental system" to underline the fact that "It has not been purposefully created but inadvertently developed" (p. 19). The U.S. health system has also been likened at times to a tremendous Rube Goldberg machine, this in reference to the American cartoonist known for his sketches of mechanical contrivances of fantastic intricacy and gadgetry.

Problem identification and assessment are basic ingredients of the policy process. When a president focuses on an issue the way Barack Obama has focused on health care, he effectively embraces the job of problem-definer in chief (Rochefort and Cobb 1994). It becomes his task to communicate the system's problems while explaining their menacing consequences. In September of 2009, President Obama delivered a nationally televised address before Congress to gather public support behind his final push for health care reform (Obama 2009). According to the *New York Times*, it was his "most forceful case yet for a sweeping health care overhaul that has eluded Washington for generations" (Stolberg and Zeleny 2009). An eloquent statement of factual analysis and moral concern on the highest level, one could hardly find a more relevant guide for taking inventory of major ills within U.S. health care.

As we have seen, scope of insurance coverage is a primary consideration when distinguishing health care across nations. In his speech, President Obama highlighted the lack of **universality** in the United States: "We are the only democracy—the only advanced democracy on Earth—the only wealthy nation—that allows such hardship for millions of its people." The president approximated that "more than 30 million American citizens ... cannot get coverage," and one of every three Americans finds himself or herself without health insurance at some point over a two-year period. Striking as these figures may be, it was an understatement of the problem. For example, latest information from the U.S. Census Bureau (2010) that is not confined to citizens alone puts the **uninsured** at nearly 51 million in 2009. This is 16.7 percent of the population. As Figure 2.1 shows, the count of uninsured has climbed sharply over the past decade with only occasional downward blips along the way.

"But the problem that plagues the health care system is not just a problem for the uninsured." Here the president was accenting the issue of coverage that fails to protect adequately against the costs of care, or that is selective with respect to illnesses for which it can be used, a plight experienced by the "**underinsured**." President Obama spoke powerfully about this growing trend:

> Those who do have insurance have never had less stability and security than they do today. More and more Americans pay their premiums, only to discover that their insurance company has dropped their coverage when they get sick, or won't pay the full cost of care. It happens every day.

Next, the president took up the concern of cost, again choosing to frame the U.S. predicament comparatively: "We spend one and a half times more per person on

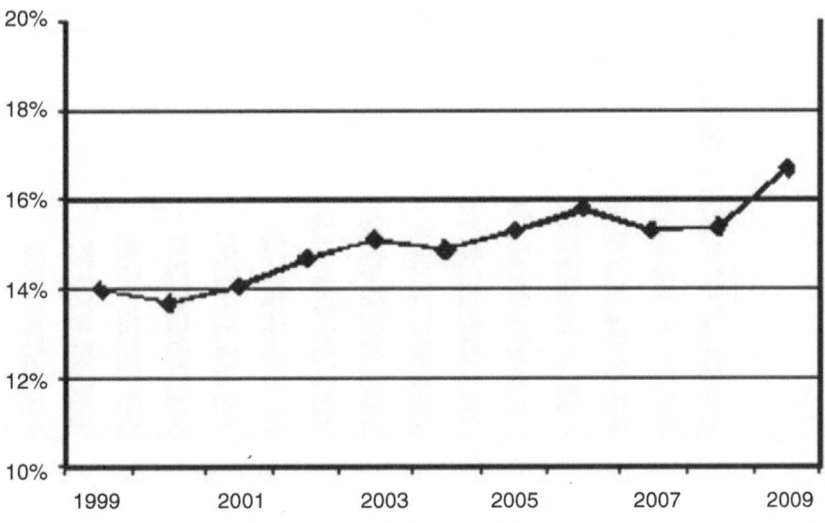

Figure 2.1 Uninsurance Rates 1999–2009

health care than any other country, but we aren't any healthier for it. This is one of the reasons that insurance premiums have gone up three times faster than wages." Now at more than 17 percent of GDP, **national health expenditures** have grown to consume more and more of the national economy since tracking figures were first published in 1929. Viewing current information cross-nationally, such as Figure 2.2 displays for OECD member nations, it is plain how much of an outlier we have become (OECD 2011).

Falling numbers of insured, eroding coverage, rising costs—each of these symptoms of an ailing system has profound implications for individuals and for society as a whole. President Obama enumerated several of the most important. Lack of coverage results in untimely delays in treatment and lack of access to needed care. The consequence, in many cases, is serious illness or avoidable death. The president told of a woman from Texas who "was about to get a double mastectomy when her insurance company canceled her policy because she forgot to declare a case of acne. By the time she had her insurance reinstated, her breast cancer had more than doubled in size." He also cited an Illinois man who "lost his coverage in the middle of chemotherapy because his insurer found that he hadn't reported gallstones that he didn't even know about." The president went further, stating the man had died from delays in treatment. In fact, the *Wall Street Journal* followed up on this anecdote and determined the individual had been able to get his insurance policy reinstated with the help of the Illinois Attorney General (Weisman 2009). This regulatory intervention did secure for him a stem-cell transplant and, as a result, the patient did not die until nearly four years later.

Rising costs also have economic effects that ripple far and wide. Today the majority of personal bankruptcies are linked to medical expenses (Himmelstein et al. 2009).

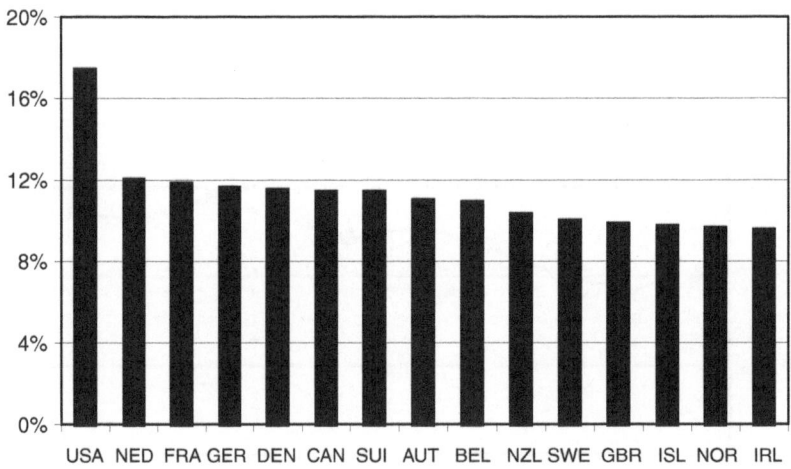

Figure 2.2 Health Spending as Percent of GDP, 2009

The president cited this financial risk, underscoring "These are not primarily people on welfare. These are middle-class Americans." He also talked about escalating premiums as the reason why "aspiring entrepreneurs cannot afford to open a business in the first place," while large "American businesses that compete internationally—like our automakers—are at a huge disadvantage." And he bemoaned the increasing expense of government health programs: "Put simply, our health care problem is our deficit problem. Nothing else even comes close. Nothing else."

Do Pieces and Parts Make a Whole?

All in all, it is a sobering catalog of inequities and inefficiencies. The next section will discuss legislation enacted by the president and his Democratic supporters based on this searing analysis of the status quo. But, first, what kind of system produces extremes of this magnitude, such professional and institutional excellence, on the one hand, matched with neglect of those in need and bloated costs, on the other? If no one designed the system to be as it is, what kinds of policies and programs sustain the established contours of U.S. health care?

Foreign observers often perceive the United States to be a bastion of private medicine without government involvement in the provision or financing of care (Peters 2004). This is a misconception. In fact, the U.S. system is a hybrid of private and public systems with several components resembling programs found elsewhere in the world. Contrary to attempts to pigeonhole U.S. health care, journalist T. R. Reid (2009) notes that "For most working people under sixty-five, we're Germany, or France, or Japan ... For Native Americans, military personnel, and veterans, we're Britain, or Cuba ... For those over sixty-five, we're Canada ... [and] For the 45 million uninsured Americans, we're Cambodia, or Burkina Faso, or rural India" (p. 20). Those who are served by federally subsidized community health centers receive their health care in a manner resembling the operation of some National Health Services.

The bedrock of U.S. health care is employment-based insurance. Of 254 million Americans with health coverage in 2009, 77 percent had private insurance, and of this amount nearly 9 in 10 got coverage through their (or a family member's) place of work, usually with premium sharing between employee and employer (U.S. Census Bureau 2010). Development of employment-based insurance as the dominant mode of coverage in the United States took place with the active encouragement of public policy makers. Under federal tax law, employers can categorize contributions to health insurance as a business expense, while the value of premiums is excluded from a worker's taxable income. During World War II, fringe benefits like health insurance also were omitted from wage controls.

No overarching public mechanism exists in the United States to rein in private health spending. Attempts to undertake system-wide population-based planning or to regulate capacity based on proven community need have not been well met by provider interests (Patel and Rushefsky 2006). During recent years, the primary effort at cost containment in private insurance is the movement known as "**managed care**," or the application of techniques of utilization review, restricted lists of providers, and payment incentives to reward cost-effective care. Managed care provoked a fierce public and professional backlash—as well as new regulatory controls over the industry—which forced insurers to backpedal (Rochefort 2001). What followed was a trend toward increased consumer cost-sharing through **deductibles**, **copayments**, and benefit reductions (Robinson 2002). Significantly, the number of companies offering health plans has also declined. In 2009, the proportion of Americans receiving coverage through work fell to its lowest level since 1987 (U.S. Census Bureau 2010). For a country reliant on the employment sector as the mainstay of health insurance coverage, it was a disquieting fact.

In 1965, the U.S. Congress adopted **Medicare**. At a time when political support for more inclusive measures was absent, it made sense for government to guarantee insurance coverage for a population group considered specially needy and sympathetic (Marmor 2000). The elderly make up the bulk of Medicare's enrollees, along with people living with certain disabilities and all persons suffering from end-stage renal disease (permanent kidney failure). In 2009, Medicare covered 46 million people, and spending totaled $509 billion (CMS 2010b). Funding is provided primarily through payroll taxes, although enrollees must contribute directly for optional benefits.

Medicare is a program of parts that has gained important facets over time, the government acting like a homeowner who adds new additions to a starter house as resources and growing ambition decide. The original law included Part A, hospital and skilled nursing care, and Part B, physician and outpatient services. In 1997, Medicare beneficiaries were given the option to enroll in Part C, private Medicare + Choice plans that offer additional benefits, like prescription drugs, vision, and dental, under various managed care and fee-for-service delivery models. Medicare Part D, made available in 2006, is a voluntary prescription drug benefit plan.

When first proposed, Medicare faced withering attacks from organized medicine, which equated it with **socialism**. Yet the program's design actually reflects a commitment to disturb private interests as little as possible. At the outset, it was decided Medicare would rely on insurance companies as administrative intermediaries while paying physicians their "usual and customary" fees and reimbursing hospitals on the basis of costs. This included generous allowance for depreciation of facilities and equipment and medical training. Eventually, open-ended payment practices of this type proved unsustainable, leading to Medicare's implementation of a prospective payment system for hospitals based on patient diagnosis in 1983, a "relative value scale" formula for physician reimbursement in 1989, and other adjustments. Even so, the federal government has always shrunk from wielding the kind of leverage in the health care market that Medicare's size would allow (Marmor and Oberlander 1998). Addition of a major drug benefit to Medicare without meaningful cost controls over the profit-driven pharmaceutical industry remains bitterly controversial.

During recent years, a number of advocates have claimed an enlargement of Medicare represents the easiest route to universal coverage and cost containment in U.S. health care (Reagan 1999; Schlesinger and Hacker 2007). Meanwhile, the latest recommendation from the political right is increased privatization of the program. It is the kind of polar contradiction that bedevils attempts to develop coherent national health policy in this country.

The other large public health insurance program in the U.S. is **Medicaid**. Like Medicare, Medicaid was created in 1965 as part of Lyndon Johnson's Great Society. However, Medicaid was less another foothold in the ascent toward full-blown national health insurance than a tactical concession by opponents to make that ascent unlikely (Marmor 2000). By 2009, Medicaid covered some 50 million people with expenditures of $381 billion—$251 billion by the federal government, and $130 billion by the states (CMS 2010a). Often, the clientele of Medicaid has been stigmatized as "welfare" recipients. This comment is not only harsh and unfair, but also less than fully accurate. Although Medicaid is a benefit received by enrollees of federal public assistance programs, many other low-income individuals and families fit the eligibility criteria. In addition, Medicaid includes large numbers of elderly recipients. In fact, long-term care takes up roughly a third of program spending nationwide.

Medicaid is a joint federal–state partnership. States enjoy considerable autonomy in administering their own programs—some provide expansive coverage and benefit options, while others are much more restrictive—but all must conform to basic federal guidelines to receive matching dollars. Federal contributions to Medicaid vary by state depending on per capita income. Changes in Medicaid over time show the same piecemeal pattern exhibited under Medicare, i.e., a series of gradual modifications broadening the program's original intent. Most important, Congress in 1997 created the **State Children's Health Insurance Program**, known commonly as CHIP, as a complement to the Medicaid program (Brandon, Chaudry, and Sardell 2001). CHIP covers uninsured children of low-income families who earn too much to qualify for Medicaid. In 2010, nearly 8 million children were covered under state CHIP programs, either through an expansion of Medicaid, creation of a separate child health program, or a combination of approaches (CMS 2010c).

Taking into account not only administrative and funding responsibilities under Medicaid, but also other activities ranging from public health services, to health facilities licensing and regulation, to medical education, it is evident states play a vital role in the U.S. health system. They also function as "laboratories" for experimenting with new policy solutions to common problems, according to the famous metaphor of Justice Louis Brandeis. So it was that over the past decade, several states moved aggressively toward comprehensive health reform while the issue languished on the national political agenda. Massachusetts adopted landmark legislation in 2006 that achieved near-universal coverage while building on the employment-based model (McDonough et al. 2006). It also introduced into mainstream health policy discourse two relatively unfamiliar programmatic concepts—the "**individual mandate**" and the "**health insurance exchange**." Both would become pillars of President Obama's health care overhaul.

Health Policy Breakthrough

Bolstered by high public approval ratings and Democratic majorities in both houses of Congress, President Obama moved quickly on his number one domestic policy initiative upon entering the Oval Office. Despite a carefully formulated political strategy, however, the push for health reform soon devolved into a contentious debate marked by partisan discord, raucous town hall meetings, and unusual legislative maneuvering. Eking out a narrow victory, President Obama signed the Patient Protection and Affordable Care Act (ACA) into law on March 23, 2010. At a ceremony in the East Room of the White House, he offered this reflection: "After a century of striving, after a year of debate, after a historic vote, health care reform is no longer an unmet promise. It is the law of the land" (Obama 2010).

The law has an implementation horizon of several years with final changes delayed until 2015, although several groups began benefiting almost immediately. For anyone still trying to keep a scorecard, there is one sense, at least, in which the U.S. stands without peer amid the international panorama of health care, and that is the multi-faceted character of its health policy solutions. This latest law is no exception (Patient Protection and Affordable Care Act 2010; see, also, Staff of *The Washington Post* 2010; White House 2010; Kaiser Family Foundation 2011a).

Within six months of the law's passage, young adults became able to remain under their parents' insurance policies up to age 26, while Medicare recipients began to receive assistance with paying for drugs under Part D, the latter a step toward eventual bigger discounts and savings meant to close coverage gaps in this benefit area. New prohibitions ended insurers' practice of denying coverage for **pre-existing conditions** for children, as well as the use of lifetime spending caps to limit selected forms of care. All new policies must now also cover specified preventive services without charging patients out-of-pocket costs. A new tax credit helps small businesses to afford coverage for employees.

Perhaps the most prominent—and widely contested—feature of the Affordable Care Act is its individual mandate. Beginning in 2014, all U.S. citizens and legal residents will be required to have health insurance or else pay a fine. However, the law makes room for "hardship exemptions" if the lowest cost plan should exceed a maximum percent of income.

Also by 2014, the law requires creation of state "exchanges" from which individuals and small businesses will be able to purchase health insurance. These bodies, administered by either a government or non-profit entity, will make it easier for those eligible to find an affordable plan while shopping a range of options. Sliding-scale subsidies will go to those purchasing insurance through an exchange whose incomes fall below 400 percent of the federal poverty level. An estimated 24 million people will get coverage through an exchange by 2018, most receiving financial assistance.

Large employers—those with 50 workers or more—face their own mandate under the law. If a business in this category fails to offer insurance coverage, or offers a plan so meager that employees end up receiving subsidies for more adequate protection from an exchange, the federal government will impose a financial penalty.

The Affordable Care Act will also expand health coverage through dramatic growth in Medicaid. All individuals under age 65 with incomes up to 133 percent of the poverty level will become eligible for the program in 2014. For newly eligible beneficiaries, an estimated 16 million people, the federal government will pay the full cost for two years. Also, beginning in 2015, states gain a substantial increase in federal funding for children's health insurance programs. Together these increases mark a conspicuous expansion in the federal government's financing of health care.

The Affordable Care Act will have significant impact on the private health insurance industry. In addition to changes already noted, as of 2014 insurers will no longer be able to turn away any applicant due to a pre-existing condition or impose limits on annual benefits. Further, beginning in 2011, insurers will be required to spend a minimum amount of premium dollars on medical services, or else send out rebates to customers.

The law contains other provisions to keep costs down. New federal rules will promote reduced paperwork through electronic record keeping. With regard to Medicare, an Independent Payment Advisory Board will report to Congress on methods for linking hospital payments to treatment effectiveness and quality. Physician payments will be shifted to take into account the "value" of care provided, not just volume.

Recognizing its potential role in improving quality and controlling costs, the law supports primary care in a variety of ways. This includes funding for training of primary care doctors, nurses, and physician assistants, as well as incentives for the creation of Accountable Care Organizations to better coordinate care received by Medicare patients served by multiple medical providers. More than $10 billion in funding for Community Health Centers is projected to nearly double the number of low-income, uninsured, minority, and other disadvantaged people served through this source. At the other end of the spectrum, the ACA also created a new long-term care insurance program for the elderly and disabled. However, this initiative has since been abandoned, due to the Administration's realization that its voluntary system of financing would likely not prove sustainable in the long run (Pear 2011).

According to the Congressional Budget Office, the health law should cost about $938 billion over the next 10 years. Financing comes, in part, from new taxes, including an excise tax on high-end "Cadillac" health plans and an increase in the Medicare payroll tax for higher-income earners. Under Medicare, payments to Part C Advantage plans will be reduced, while hospitals and other institutional providers will receive smaller increases in their payment rates. New annual fees on the pharmaceutical and health insurance industries, as well as penalties collected from individuals and employers who violate coverage mandates, constitute other major sources of financing.

Of Wish Lists and Uncertain Outcomes

The new health law is perhaps best described as a collection of patches, stopgaps, and redirections meant to counter the existing system's most obvious dysfunctions while extending benefits to more of the population. It represents a very pragmatic approach, politically and programmatically, to the issues itemized by the president. One might be tempted to re-label the bill the American Health System Preservation Act, given its careful avoidance of large-scale restructuring of the health sector. The question is, does the law do enough?

Among the most obvious exclusions from the health law is the "public option." This catchphrase refers to a proposal to offer government-sponsored insurance alongside private health plans within the new exchanges. In his speech of September 2009, the president spoke at length about the public option, stating forcefully that it would put "pressure on private insurers to keep their policies affordable and treat their customers better." Many liberal Democrats insisted it was indispensable. The insurance industry stood opposed (together with other institutional interests and some centrist Democrats) and won the day.

Nor does the Affordable Care Act promise universal coverage. The Congressional Budget Office estimates 23 million people will remain uninsured by 2019—almost a full decade after the law's adoption. About seven million will be undocumented immigrants. Additional uninsured will include people eligible for Medicaid benefits who do not enroll, and those who choose to absorb the tax penalty rather than buy mandatory health insurance (Mertens 2010). The size of this latter group hinges on the affordability of options under the new law, as does the scope of the population that qualifies for exemption from the insurance mandate.

Thus is cost containment critical to this law's success, although in no respect is there more uncertainty about the president's program. According to Obama advisors Peter Orszag and Ezekiel Emanuel (2010), the law "puts into place virtually every cost-control reform proposed by physicians, economists, and health policy experts and includes the means for these reforms to be assessed quickly and scaled up if they're successful" (p. 603). Yet critics on both left and right cast doubt on projected cost savings so heavily dependent on future action by Congress (Holtz-Eakin and Ramlet 2010). Further, because of political concessions made during the legislative process, the Affordable Care Act effectively directs millions of new subscribers to private insurers without either accompanying price controls or external competition.

Conclusion

The Affordable Care Act marks a watershed in U.S. health policy, but it is no end point. Leading Republicans did not even wait for ink on the bill to dry before vowing repeal. Implementation challenges under the law are huge as states face the job of instituting new insurance exchanges, ramping up for Medicaid expansion, and managing new administrative assignments, all with limited bureaucratic capacity at a time of fiscal distress. The federal government must coordinate this far-flung undertaking. Tom Daschle, former Democratic Senate Majority Leader and informal health care advisor to President Obama, put it best when commenting that passage of the law was not a "touchdown." Rather, "we are only on the thirty-yard line, with seventy yards left to go" (Daschle 2010: 264). Moving the ball farther down field, reformers will need to fashion a playbook filled with many options. The remainder of this book looks abroad as one rich source of experience for this endeavor.

DISCUSSION QUESTIONS

1. What has been your personal experience with the U.S. health care system? How have you encountered the benefits and/or drawbacks associated with its unique "patchwork" design?
2. Are you impressed or dismayed by the tendency within U.S. health policy to maximize the pluralism of the health sector by maintaining an array of different private and public programs?
3. Which aspects of the Affordable Care Act do you believe are likely to bring the greatest improvements to U.S. health care? What parts of the law would you like to see changed?
4. All things considered, do you think U.S. leaders followed the best possible path in their approach to health reform?

III: Health and Society

"Fish would be the last to discover water." This proverb offers a pithy reminder about how easy it is to lose sight of things with which we are most familiar. The challenge of self-awareness arises for anyone wanting to understand issues of health and health care policy. Culture, social structure, the distribution of resources—all are powerful forces shaping national health systems, yet their impact is so pervasive they blend unnoticed into the deep background of our lives. Health policy is not made in a vacuum. A macro view of the intersection between health and society highlights the communal factors underlying public demands and government choices in this realm. It also calls attention to the bold interventions adopted by some other countries in tackling the social origins of illness and wellbeing.

Thinking about Culture and Health

A seemingly inexhaustible source of theorizing and applied research, **culture** is truly one of the "big ideas" of social science (Quah 2010). The famous anthropologist Clyde Kluckhohn once counted more than 150 definitions of culture. This list continues to grow. Kluckhohn himself favored the pleasingly terse formulation of culture as a community's "design for living" based on "patterned ways of thinking, feeling, and reacting" (quoted in Quah 2010: 29).

Culture is a concept of obvious importance in the study of health systems (Helman 2007). First, a nation's culture refers to its collective identity growing out of the population's shared history, institutions, beliefs, and social values. Second, culture is also a variable sensitive to heterogeneity *within* national boundaries to the extent that particular groups possess distinctive experiences and outlooks.

Cultural predispositions not only contribute to behaviors that reduce or lessen the likelihood of disease, they also condition perceptions of what disease is, how individuals respond to the experience of illness, and the types of treatments expected from a system of care. For medical sociologists, these are well-known facts. As David Mechanic concluded more than three decades ago, "Cultures are so recognizably different that variations in illness behavior in different societies hardly need demonstration" (quoted in Quah 2010: 35). Similarly, the practice of medicine, which both shapes and responds to patient preferences, cannot be understood apart from cultural context. On the plane of service infrastructure, health system organization within Western societies has been driven by the relationship between biomedical science and technological advancement, on the one hand, and popular and professional support for the innovations they bring, on the other (Mechanic and Rochefort 1996).

Surprising discrepancies exist in the way physicians from different countries assess cause of death when viewing the same death certificates. Numbers and types of symptoms of psychiatric patients, as well as their diagnostic interpretation, can depend on the nationality of mental health clinicians. Treatments viewed as helpful in some societies—homeopathic remedies, spa visits, approved prescription drugs—are ignored, or recommended much less frequently, in others. Nations even betray varying preoccupations with particular organs as sites of disease. The French demonstrate ingrained interest in the liver; Germans devote particular attention to the heart. For its part, American medicine stands out for aggressive use of expensive diagnostic tests and a propensity for surgical intervention. As summarized by the researcher who compiled this information: "The array of viable medical traditions certainly suggests that medicine is not the international science many think it is. Indeed, it may never be. Medical research can indicate the likely consequences of a given course of action, but any decision about whether those consequences are desirable must first pass through the filter of cultural values" (Payer 1990: 42; see also, Payer 1988).

In his recent investigation of health care in France, Germany, Japan, the United Kingdom, and Canada, T. R. Reid (2009) conducted a personal experiment in comparative medical evaluation by speaking with physicians in each country about a nagging shoulder ailment. This series of consultations yielded a dizzying spectrum of treatment advice: major surgery, steroid injections, physical therapy, acupuncture, even stoic endurance. In this way one author's physical complaint sampled the behavior of entire systems of care, revealing the coincidence of cultural values, clinical judgment, and resource prioritization in health care delivery. Simply to record such divergent patterns is to acknowledge the reality of options in health system design.

The Politics–Culture Connection

Different dimensions of culture come into play in different arenas of society. According to one durable description, **political culture** is "the set of attitudes, beliefs, and sentiments which give order and meaning to a political process and which provide the underlying assumptions and rules that govern behavior in the political system" (Pye 1968: 218). Both ideals and operational realities, the orientations of citizens as well as their leaders, are embraced by this term. Although the content of political culture is never constant from one society to another, certain themes or functions are universal, among them the following:

1. Setting the boundary between public and private sectors.
2. Determining the legitimate scope and uses of public authority.
3. Cultivating citizen identification with the polity.
4. Building trust in the structures of government decision making.

One misconception is that a focus on political culture implies lack of change. While established loyalties, reinforced by customary ways of thinking and doing, may promote stability, political cultures everywhere must allow for problem solving and resolution of grievances. Core values themselves can shift within nations, the result of novel events and experiences, a cultural trait of adaptability, and large-scale socioeconomic trauma (Eckstein 1988). Further, the link between political culture and policy choice runs in more than one direction. How new laws and programs perform has potential for altering the way citizens see their government, and established social relations can be redirected under influence of law. These latter points are worth keeping in mind in regard to arguments about the fundamental incompatibility between health policies in foreign countries and American culture.

If political culture helps account for resistance to change, it also casts light on how systems cope when circumstances make change inevitable. In an earlier time, national policy frameworks arranging health care for all elements of the population would have been unthinkable. If inertia were a fixed rule in politics, the matter would have ended there. However, since Germany's first tentative steps with the Health Insurance Bill of 1883 under Chancellor Bismarck, national health insurance and its variants have increasingly become the norm in economically advanced societies. This is so even in the United States, which zigzags ever closer to making health care security a guaranteed fact under law.

"[E]ach country brings to health a distinctive combination of historical and cultural factors that are crucial in explaining its proclivities and characteristics," write Robert Blank and Viola Burau (2010: 45). Of primary concern for these scholars are norms governing the relationship between individuals and society as a whole. Some nations, like Germany, The Netherlands, and Japan, have "communitarian" political cultures centering on the interests of defined communities based on demographic, geographic, and other criteria. Others, like Sweden, New Zealand, and the United Kingdom, are more "egalitarian" in their commitment to social welfare benefits as entitlements for all. A third grouping of nations, which includes the U.S., Australia, and Singapore, is "individualistic" in that individual liberties often take priority over collective interests. This template justifies neither rigid policy predictions, nor the neglect of telling eccentricities within individual political systems. Nonetheless, it is an intriguing framework for contemplating culture and health care from a comparative perspective, including the use of public and private programs, government regulation, and issues of cost and access.

Two Examples

Two areas of contemporary medicine illustrate the role of cultural factors in health care. They also show how difficult it is to decouple the umbrella of culture from a society's politics and economics.

Our first example is the problem of psychological **depression**. Whereas **anxiety** was the most diagnosed and treated mental health condition among Americans in the post-World War II era, today that position has been taken over by depression (Horwitz 2010). Underlying this shift are growth trends nothing short of remarkable. Between 1987 and 1997, the proportion of the population receiving outpatient treatment for depression increased 300 percent. By 2002, depression accounted for more than three times as many outpatient visits as anxiety. A landmark international survey of mental disorders was carried out in 2001–2003 (WHO World Mental Health Consortium 2004). It found that, among 14 developed and undeveloped countries studied, the U.S. had the highest rate of depression and related mood disorders. Use of **antidepressants** has risen in tandem with diagnosis and services utilization, making these medications the largest selling category of all drugs inside the U.S. More than one in ten members of the population now take antidepressants, and the trend is upward (Szabo 2009).

What accounts for the arrival of this "age of depression," in Allan Horwitz's (2010) evocative phrase? A comprehensive answer may be elusive, but several causes are evident. More precise diagnostic criteria for depression emerged within the field of psychiatry. As part of their growing interest in biologically based conditions, researchers and psychiatric professionals steered attention to depression, with mental health advocacy groups following suit. Expanded information about depressive conditions, combined with the instrumental appeal of new medications, boosted the public's willingness to seek treatment.

Yet this list of explanations is inadequate if corporate and governmental behaviors are omitted. In office-based psychiatry brief medication consultations have become standard while in-depth counseling is rapidly disappearing (Harris 2011). The reason is simple. Insurance industry policies discourage lengthy therapy sessions by means of low reimbursement rates and a narrowing of the concept of "medically necessary" treatment. Also relevant to the popularity of antidepressants is medical advertising. Pharmaceutical companies spend billions each year "selling the disease of depression," in addition to specific drugs, to the public and medical practitioners (Horwitz 2010: 130; Donohue, Cevasco, and Rosenthal 2007). As one critic of the industry has observed, "by the late 1980s, the pharmaceutical industry's storytelling apparatus had evolved into a well-oiled machine" (Whitaker 2010: 254). The U.S. government facilitated this marketing assault when the Food and Drug Administration loosened regulatory policies in the late 1990s to allow television advertising of prescription drugs targeted directly at consumers. In 2002, investigators from the U.S. General Accounting Office found that consumer advertising increased nearly 150 percent following the revised regulations. The agency estimated 8.5 million Americans requested and received prescriptions for drugs after seeing or hearing ads for those products, some of which included false or misleading information (Pear 2002).

At present, the situation stands as follows. Substantial numbers of people suffering from depression do not receive treatment, while many people taking antidepressants fail to meet the diagnostic criteria for them. At the same time, there is mounting research that raises questions about the efficacy of antidepressants compared to **placebos** or to **psychotherapy** as a treatment alternative (Antonuccio, Burns, and Danton 2002). All in all, it is an odd "model of care" to export to other countries, but that is effectively what large American (and British) drug manufacturers are doing via aggressive product marketing of antidepressants in South America, India, Japan, and elsewhere abroad.

Public health experts have cited the need for more robust monitoring of the safety of antidepressants in the U.S. following the example of surveillance systems already in place in other countries (Busch and Barry 2009). Britain's National Institute for Health and Clinical Excellence, a special independent authority set up within the National Health Service, disseminated clinical guidelines for the treatment and management of depression that included the following caution: "Do not use antidepressants routinely to treat persistent subthreshold depressive symptoms or mild depression because the risk-benefit ratio is poor" (NICE 2009: 21).

A more wholesale approach to reform, and one fully in keeping with the 2010 Affordable Care Act, whose Section 5604 calls for demonstration projects in this area, would be to improve integration of mental health services within **primary care** settings. Here again, foreign nations may have something to show the United States. A 2008 report by the World Health Organization presented detailed descriptions of integration programs in Argentina, Australia, South Africa, Belize, Brazil, Saudi Arabia, and other locales around the world. Service structures and financing approaches differ, and close examination is needed to evaluate which examples might be most workable in the U.S. health policy environment. Yet, in general, all attest to the potential for "closing the treatment gap," as well as "ensuring that people get the mental health care they need," by instituting formal collaboration among specialists, general practitioners, auxiliary caregivers, and providers of community-based services (WHO and Wonca 2008: 1).

Our second example is the problem of **obesity**. Although obesity has been a public health concern for decades, today it is considered an **epidemic** with far-reaching impacts on population health (Visscher and Seidell 2001). Obesity is associated with a range of chronic health conditions, including heart disease, cancer, muscular-skeletal disorders, respiratory disorders, and type 2 diabetes. For this reason, obesity is a major risk factor in premature death, **morbidity**, and **disability**, its contribution to the burden of disease now comparable to smoking, that long-time nemesis of the public health community (Jia and Lubetkin 2010). According to the U.S. Centers for Disease Control and Prevention, direct and indirect costs of obesity approximate 10 percent of national health expenditures in the United States (Finkelstein et al. 2009).

Latest estimates are that one-third of the adult U.S. population is obese; this figure reaches 68 percent for obesity and **overweight** combined (Flegal et al. 2010). Obesity is a global health problem. Increases are greatest in developed countries, but numbers have been trending up in developing countries as well. Nonetheless, when viewed along the international continuum, American obesity rates fall at the extreme high end. In a recent report by the OECD (2010), among more than 30 nations considered, the U.S. had the highest percentage of obese and overweight adults. When the CDC compared obesity rates between the U.S. and Canada, the U.S. topped its northern neighbor by more than 10 percent (Shields, Carroll, and Ogden 2011). As one commentator marveled, not even "all the poutine (cheese curds, gravy and fries) in Quebec and Tim Hortons' doughnut shops from coast to coast" could put Canadians on a par with Americans (Hensley 2011).

Cultural factors are integral to the obesity picture. A sedentary lifestyle has evolved in the United States (Agger 2010). Physical activity is declining due to changing types of work, and levels of recreational exercise remain low (Brownson, Boehmer, and Luke 2005). Suburban living induces dependence on the automobile. Even the number of children walking or bicycling to school is down sharply from earlier decades. The Nielsen Company (2009) reported television watching at an all-time high for the 2008–2009 television season: an average of 4 hours and 49 minutes per person (2 years and over) per day. Potato chips and French fries account for nearly one-quarter of all vegetable servings consumed by American children (Schlosser 2005: 241).

Individualism, liberty, and laissez-faire are basic values within the American creed that militate against activist government and encourage personal responsibility for one's behavior (Lipset 1996). But there is a "political economy of obesity" that can only be addressed by public policy. Public policies, or their absence, are critical in determining the food environment within which eating choices are made. "[G]overnment policies regarding such issues as agricultural subsidies and dietary guidance, as well as industry influence through food advertising and the production of highly processed, low-nutrition foods, comprise factors with which individuals cannot alone cope," writes Suzanne Havala Hobbs, Professor of Public Health at the University of Carolina at Chapel Hill. "Behind these issues are myriad influential interests, many of which stand to lose should substantial and effective steps be taken toward remedies by local, state or provincial or national governments" (Hobbs 2008: 9).

Earlier a parallel was noted concerning the impacts of obesity and smoking on the health status of the population. It seems only fitting, then, that policy analysts have begun to propose strategies to reduce obesity based on tobacco-control tactics. A 2008 advisory by the Urban Institute pointed to the following categories of action:

new taxes on fattening food of little nutritional value; clear labeling on the front of packaged foods to show their nutritional content; requirements on restaurant chains to include nutritional information throughout their menus; and banning advertising and limiting the marketing of fattening food (Engelhard, Garson, and Dorn 2009).

Part "think tank" and part "advocacy group," the International Obesity Task Force (IOTF) combats obesity on the global stage. In August of 2010, the IOTF convened an international congress in Sweden to review "the progress countries were making in instituting effective, sustainable policies for the prevention of obesity" (IOTF 2010: 2). Two nations won honors as international leaders on this issue, England and Brazil, whose model practices and policies included sophisticated surveillance of obesity trends, tough food marketing regulation, improved school meal programs, incorporation of obesity prevention and management as priority national health policy goals, and more.

To be sure, the U.S. has its own plethora of anti-obesity initiatives. Yet programs and laws vary tremendously from state to state, while the federal government mostly confines itself to research and education efforts (and paying for obesity-related illnesses through Medicare and Medicaid). Despite promising new approaches, the 2010 edition of *F as in Fat*, a comprehensive report by Trust for America's Future and the Robert Wood Johnson Foundation, assigned a very low grade to America's obesity policies: "[O]ur response as a nation has yet to fully match the magnitude of the problem" (p. 3). Was it more culture or politics that led Sarah Palin, former Governor of Alaska and vice-presidential candidate, to complain that First Lady Michelle Obama's "Let's Move" fitness campaign threatened her and her countrymen's "God-given rights to make our own decisions" (Katz 2010)? Whatever the answer may be for this **populist** "hockey mom," Palin's statement gives voice to the resistance sure to be met by more resolute government action in the fight against obesity in our society.

Does Society Make us Sick?

In 2008 a child born in Afghanistan or Zimbabwe, the countries at the bottom of the world's **life expectancy** distribution, could expect to live 42 years on average. One born in Japan or San Marino, the countries at the top, could expect to live 83 years (WHO 2010b). Extremes in **infant mortality rate**, another key vital statistic that counts deaths by age 1 per 1,000 live births, range from 165 in Afghanistan to 1 in San Marino and 2 in Iceland, Luxembourg, Singapore, Slovenia, and Sweden. People between the ages of 15 and 60 face a .772 probability of dying in Zimbabwe, compared to a probability of .053 in San Marino and .056 in Iceland. Paralleling such differences *among* countries are stark differences *within*. In the United States in 2006, infant mortality rate was 13.35 per 1,000 live births for Black Americans, and 5.58 per 1,000 live births for Whites. It was almost as if the former racial group lived in Albania (IMR=13), while the latter lived in New Zealand (IMR=5).

Table 3.1 Comparative Health Measures

	Life Expectancy from Birth 2008	Infant Mortality 2008 (deaths during first year of life per 1,000 live births)	Adult Mortality 2008 (probability of dying between 15 and 60 years of age per 1,000 population)
Afghanistan	42		
Zimbabwe	42		
Japan	83		
San Marino	83		
United States	78		
Afghanistan		165	
San Marino		1	
Iceland		2	
Luxembourg		2	
Singapore		2	
Slovenia		2	
Sweden		2	
United States		7	
Zimbabwe			772
San Marino			53
Iceland			56
United States			107

Source: World Health Organization, World Health Statistics 2010 (2010b).

As the biologist Stephen Jay Gould (1985) has written, variation is "nature's only irreducible essence." The simple fact of measured differences in health is not surprising. What is remarkable, however, are two characteristics of this variation. One is the sheer amount of inequality that exists—for some indicators as much as a full order of magnitude. The other is the fact that these differences are neither random nor fixed. Rather, they are "systematic" (exhibiting reliable patterns across socioeconomic strata), "socially produced" (resulting from social rather than biological processes), and "unfair" (giving certain groups a higher possibility of survival and thriving than others) (Whitehead and Dahlgren 2007).

Growing awareness of these facts, matched with a concern for social justice and human rights, has spurred a vigorous international research agenda under the rubric of "**social determinants of health**." Whereas populations (and individuals) possess inherent biological and genetic traits, health is also produced by a collection of alterable factors. These factors operate on micro, meso, and macro levels—from individual lifestyle, to social and community factors, to living and working conditions, to general socioeconomic, cultural, and environmental conditions (see Figure 3.1).

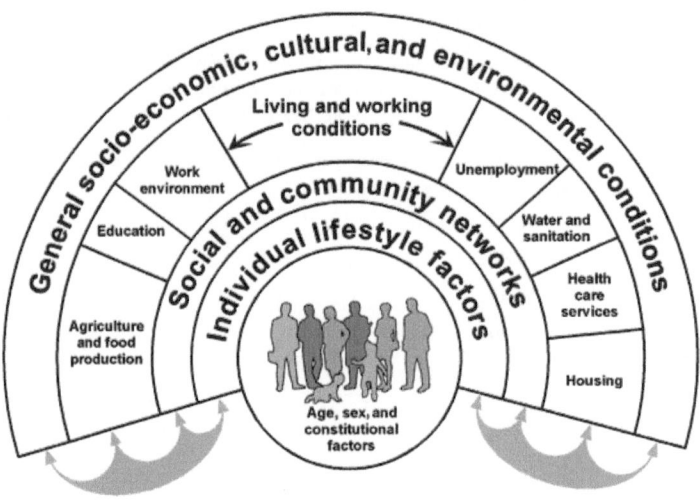

Source: Dahlgren and Whitehead, 1993, 2007

Figure 3.1 The Main Determinants of Health

In addition to its panoramic view of health as a social phenomenon, the result of "causes behind causes," this framework represents a potentially powerful tool of policy analysis by spotlighting points of leverage for shifting the status quo. In 2008, the WHO's Commission on Social Determinants of Health began its final report with these candid words: "These inequities in health, avoidable health inequalities, arise because of the circumstances in which people grow, live, work, and age, and the systems put in place to deal with illness. The conditions in which people live and die are, in turn, shaped by political, social, and economic forces" (WHO 2008: i).

Even within a complex web of influences, economic factors are paramount when it comes to health disparities. For individuals, living in poverty can interfere with satisfaction of basic needs, lead to adverse living environments, result in hazardous working conditions, be associated with unhealthy lifestyle choices, reduce educational opportunities, and limit access to health care. All elevate the risks of illness, injury, or premature death. Yet poverty's impact is not simple. It is entangled with many other variables, particularly race, in a society like the United States (Budrys 2010). Nor do economic resource levels translate neatly into health outcomes on the cross-national level. Comparing the mortality and gross national product of various countries, there are many instances where the two factors show little correlation (Marmot 2005).

A fuller understanding requires considering how available resources are distributed. The effect of socioeconomic inequality on health status is well documented, both across and inside societies. But is the culprit perceived deprivation, or an actual lack of critical resources for some groups? Sociologist Grace Budrys (2010) states how inequality qualifies the experience of poverty: "Living in a society where what you have is not that different from what others have means that you are not poor. Living in a society where some people have a great deal more than you do makes it obvious how deprived you are" (p. 198). A recent work called *The Spirit Level: Why Greater Equality Makes Societies Stronger*, by Richard Wilkinson and Kate Picket (2010), reviews myriad strands of evidence pertinent to this quandary. The research of these authors inclines them toward a "psychosocial" interpretation in which "The biology of chronic stress is a plausible pathway which helps us to understand why unequal societies are almost always unhealthy societies" (p. 87).

Health Policy Interventions Abroad

In a mode at once playful and sharply serious, the Canadian Centre for Social Justice offered several tips for better health applying the insights of social determinants research (cited in Grantmakers in Health 2007). Topping the list are these two recommendations: 1. Don't be poor. If you can, stop. If you can't, try not to be poor for long. 2. Don't have poor parents.

Assuming most individuals already agree about the desirability of not being poor and have little to say about who their parents are, how can empirical knowledge of the impact of societal factors be used to guide health policy? Or, to borrow Whitehead and Dahlgren's (2007) phrase, what "pragmatic principles of action" emerge from this field, and how can other countries instruct an American audience? Of greatest interest here are democratic, economically advanced nations, a group whose political and socioeconomic environments most closely approximate the U.S. context.

Sweden's parliament adopted a new public health policy in 2003 shifting focus from disease to health determinants (Lundgren 2009). With this reorientation came heightened attention to structural factors, living conditions, and health behaviors as the basis for long-term social action. An extensive series of indicators was compiled for monitoring, and efforts undertaken, first, to coordinate public agencies on central, regional, and county levels and, second, to assess the role of current activities in improving health determinants. This consultation raised consciousness about the influences of government across-the-board on health while prioritizing dozens of proposals for enhanced public health work. In 2006, a center–right coalition government gained power in Sweden, refocusing public health policy with an emphasis on children, the health service proper, and health-related behaviors. This development made plain the role of politics in deciding the scope of policy action on health determinants, although health equity remains intact as a fundamental objective for this nation.

Over the past 20 years, the issue of **health inequities** has risen dramatically on the political agenda in Norway. Although positive health indicators in this "social democratic" state may be the envy of most of the rest of the world, they conceal extensive differences among social groups. Following a series of white papers in the 1980s, 1990s, and 2000s detailing the problem, in 2007 a coalition government of the Labour Party, Socialist Left Party, and Center Party announced a comprehensive strategy aimed at reducing social inequalities in health. There are four priority areas: 1. Reducing inequities in income, childhood conditions, and work-life factors that contribute to differences in health; 2. Reducing inequities in health-related behaviors and health services utilization; 3. Targeting initiatives for social integration of vulnerable populations; and 4. Building a knowledge base, as well as tools, for action across multiple sectors of public administration (Dahl and Lie 2009).

In 2010, the WHO convened a meeting of senior officials and planners from a wide range of countries in Adelaide, Australia, to discuss implementation of public polices for achieving health equity. A central conclusion was the need for a "Health in All Policies Approach." As articulated in the final report of this gathering,

> The Adelaide Statement on Health in All Policies is to engage leaders and policy-makers at all levels of government—local, regional, national and international. It emphasizes that government objectives are best achieved when all sectors include health and well-being as a key component of policy development. This is because the causes of health and well-being lie outside the health sector and are socially and economically formed.
>
> (WHO 2010a: 1)

Far from some pie-in-sky abstraction, the Adelaide Statement reflects activities already under way in some nations. A good case in point is Finland (Puska and Ståhl 2010). The starting point here dates back to the 1970s, when Finnish policy makers implemented a broad national program to reduce cardiovascular disease through changes in national diet. Use of community organizations to provide preventive services and public information became a model for partnership involving government agencies and public and private sectors. The objective was nothing less than changing the "social, physical, and policy environment," including important regulatory and subsidy reforms governing agriculture and commerce. In 2006, Finland adopted a "Health in All Policies" initiative based on the success of this national nutrition effort. In addition to making this theme central to Finland's presidency of the European Union, government leaders launched a series of measures regarding health promotion, identification and reduction of health inequalities, and increased taxation of tobacco, alcohol, and unhealthy foods.

In a recent expert review of global action on the social determinants of health, the U.S. highlight was not public policy development, but rather the formation of a "Commission to Build a Healthier America" by the private Robert Wood Johnson Foundation, most of whose recommendations "focused on the individual," not broader social and economic change (Friel and Marmot 2011: 231). In 2011, the Centers for Disease

Control initiated a new publication, entitled the "Health Disparities and Inequalities Report," for the purpose of consolidating indicators relating to mortality, morbidity, behavioral risk factors, health care access, preventive services, and social determinants of critical health problems in the U.S. (Truman et al. 2011). This action caps a long span of data gathering and research grant making by the U.S. Department of Health and Human Services (HHS) and other federal agencies on this issue. The Affordable Care Act quietly extends this approach via Sec. 4302, which directs the HHS Secretary to oversee collection of demographic data relevant to health disparities under federally supported health programs. But it is one thing to document health disparities and inequalities, and quite another to overcome the political barriers that inhibit translating this information into effective policy as a matter of "distributive justice" (Gamble and Stone 2006).

The issue of inequality and its deleterious health effects is particularly nettlesome for the U.S., where political culture provides meager support for greater equality as an explicit policy goal. Indeed, income inequality in the U.S., already greatest among advanced industrialized economies, increased over the period 1997 to 2007 (Truman et al. 2011). Yet, as Wilkinson and Picket (2010) argue, many possible routes can be taken for narrowing income differences. Not all countries around the world choose **redistributive taxes**, a notion often portrayed as off-limits in contemporary American politics, although some polls do indicate substantial support for raising taxes on upper-income earners if it would otherwise mean cutting health programs or increasing the deficit (see, e.g., Thomma 2011). Alternatives include corporate tax reform, employee-shared management and ownership of companies, minimum wage updates, broader distribution of new technologies such as Internet access, and enhanced access to higher education. One valuable lesson from Norway is the importance of universal benefits as a means of avoiding stigmatizing those most helped by social welfare policies (Dahl and Lie 2009). The challenge, then, is not so much lack of information about what might be done, but rather summoning political will for the task (Wilkinson and Picket 2010).

Conclusion

Health and illness are matters of individual biology, but they are also social phenomena in their meaning, occurrence, and definition as political issues. The purpose of this chapter has been to provide a framework for appreciating this reality and for examining the connection between health and society cross-nationally. Discussion has been sweeping in its overview of the field of "social medicine" and the policy options it poses for Americans. The following three chapters narrow in on law making for national health reform, beginning with the subject of politics followed by policy design and program implementation.

DISCUSSION QUESTIONS

1. How do you think your cultural background and values shape your approach to personal health and your expectations of the health care system?
2. In what ways do you think American society sends mixed messages about improving population health and following a healthy lifestyle?
3. Michelle Obama and Sarah Palin seem to have very different opinions about the role government should play in the fight against obesity. What are their points of view and with whom do you most agree?
4. Describe various ways in which "social factors" contribute to health inequities in the United States. Which health policy interventions abroad discussed in this chapter could be most helpful in this country?

IV: The Politics of Health Reform

Politics is the major obstacle to health care reform. The greatest improvements in the social organization of health care in this country have been achieved through politics. These statements seem contradictory, yet both are true. In politics, change is more the exception than the rule. Our form of government promotes stability, and the status quo always has beneficiaries who defend it mightily. Sometimes, however, a "perfect storm" of events and forces will sweep away all sources of inertia to usher in public policies of a transformative character. Tip O'Neill, legendary Speaker of the U.S. House of Representatives, famously commented: "All politics is local." A more apt motto for this book is: "All politics is global." An enduring set of dilemmas, fault lines, and likely trajectories typifies the health policy process. These elements come plainly into view cross-nationally. Although it is impossible to find another country that has traveled the exact road beckoning the United States forward, struggles from other times and places signal possibilities, as well as looming risks, in our own political situation.

A Primer on the Policy Process

Politics may be a great "spectator sport," but when it comes to law making much of the process is chaotic and poorly visible. A schematic model outlined by health policy specialist Beaufort Longest (2003) helps to bring order, in broad terms, to what goes on inside and outside of public view.

First, public policy making is an "open" process shaped by internal and external factors. The deliberative workings of government, policy preferences of officials, and budgetary realities all belong to the former category. Examples of external demands and inputs are stakeholder pressures, expert advice, and **public opinion**. As social conditions change, the need for policy action may increase or decrease. Legal decisions help to establish the context within which different policy approaches become more or less feasible.

Second, the main activities of this process cluster around certain phases. During *policy formulation*, issues gain a place on the governmental agenda and policy remedies are developed and adopted. *Policy implementation* is concerned with putting laws and programs into effect. And *policy modification* involves the assessment and possible correction or replacement of policies already in existence.

Third, public policy making is "distinctly cyclical." Decisions are rarely final; rather, they are constantly subject to revision and review. No consensus is guaranteed to last for long. This is true because the strength and alignment of political actors may be different tomorrow than it is today. Further, new information about the state of society is always coming to light, which can alter expectations of what government can and should be doing.

What distinguishes the relatively few problems that receive attention from government at any point in time? Nothing can happen until a problem gains recognition. This usually depends on high-profile incidents and fact gathering that document the injurious situation in an unmistakable way. Next, there must be agreement on a suitable solution within the capacity of government to carry out. Last, the political environment must be receptive toward policy action based on such factors as public mood, the stances of political parties and **interest groups**, and executive leadership. This framework is equally useful for examining "ideas whose time has come" and those out of sync with the moment. In fact, one of the principal case studies inspiring this analysis of converging problem, policy, and political streams was the collapse of national health insurance proposals in the late 1970s (Kingdon 1995).

Most public issues are multi-faceted and open to interpretation. This leads to competition among divergent perspectives within the policy process (Entman 2004). Should access to health care services be approached as a right of citizenship, or as a question of personal responsibility? Is the market a source of health care inequality, or a potential means for improving the distribution of health care resources? Obviously, whichever frame of reference wins out will affect the way lawmakers respond. Elected officials and other political actors often resort to symbolic and metaphorical language to build support for one policy frame over another (Stone 2001). The media are pivotal in broadcasting these rhetorical narratives about public policy issues to the general public (Gamson and Modigliani 1989).

Interest groups are endemic in the workings of government, although few policy domains possess such a profusion of well-organized interests as health care. Medical associations, health insurers, hospitals, pharmaceutical corporations, consumer alliances, businesses, and unions are just some of the hundreds of groups that lobby on health legislative issues (Weissert and Weissert 2006). Campaigns mounted by special interests are increasingly sophisticated today, involving political donations, commercial advertising, research initiatives, protest activities, and other methods of influence.

Historically, the **lobbying** activities of physician organizations in the United States have often limited government's ability to intervene in the health sector (Godt 1987). Insurers played the part of major spoiler in mobilizing against the Clinton health reform of the early 1990s. Anticipated reaction from such political heavyweights can go far in deciding the kinds of health policy proposals officials are willing to introduce. With most major interest groups devoted to protecting their stake in the existing system, the policy process is prone to "dynamics without change," that is, a stalemate among contending political stakeholders in which only moderate change is possible (Alford 1972: 140).

The United States has a great many "**policy venues**," or institutional points of decision making, across different branches of government and federal, state, and local levels (Baumgartner and Jones 1993). If the policy window is closed in one venue, it may be open in another. Advocates search for the best opportunities, or points of leverage, to pursue policy change, using success at one location and with one set of officials as a springboard for action elsewhere in the political system. For more than a century now, the issue of health insurance expansion has bounced back and forth between the federal government and the states. In this way the issue has managed to survive despite repeated institutional rebukes. Yet this same diffusion of authority affords policy opponents the chance to play venues against each other. Making its way through the court system is a challenge to the Affordable Care Act's individual mandate provision, a very significant matter that has finally landed in the hands of the U.S. Supreme Court.

Comparative policy analysis often focuses on structures of government and the opportunities and constraints they provide (see, e.g., Immergut 1992). Procedural rules controlling the way legislatures, courts, and bureaucracies function—including their agenda setting methods—vary across nations. The U.S. policy apparatus takes its form according to a framework of **checks and balances** created by the Constitution. Multiple **veto points** tend to advantage minority interests intent on defeating legislative proposals. In traditional **parliamentary systems**, law making moves more quickly, especially when strong party discipline is combined with a single party's dominating control of executive and legislative functions. Institutional differences of this kind are an important reason why universal health care systems developed in other democratic countries faster than here at home.

The Great Health Reform Battle of 2009–2010

The Affordable Care Act moved through the policy formulation stage relatively quickly, from early 2009 when President Obama put the issue of health reform at the top of the national agenda to final passage in March of 2010. The law is now more than one year into the preliminary stage of policy implementation and, sure enough, a number of modifications have come under review. These range from technical adjustments, such as a change in tax reporting requirements proposed by the Administration, to Republican efforts to dismantle the law as national policy. If we look back on the battle that gave birth to this reform, what does it reveal about the contemporary health policy process in this country?

As already noted, a problem must be matched with a feasible solution in the policy-making process. In this case, the solution was the individual mandate. Originally a conservative idea, the individual mandate gained prominence as part of a bipartisan solution to establish universal health care in Massachusetts. Republicans rebuffed it anyway on the national level. Even Mitt Romney, Massachusetts Governor at the time of the 2006 reform, rejected it as inappropriate policy for the federal government. Republicans now framed the Democratic proposal as an expensive big government plan, while maintaining that only a market-oriented system could bring meaningful change to American health care. Republicans also argued states should be free to develop their own reforms instead of having a program built around strong national standards.

As the push for reform ramped up, President Obama sought to stem the inevitable tide of interest group opposition by making certain accommodations up front. He promised to shield the pharmaceutical industry from additional controls in return for an $80 billion pledge to lower the cost of prescription drugs. This deal, wrote the *New York Times*, offered "a window on the secretive and potentially risky game the Obama administration has played … to line up support from industry groups typically hostile to government health care initiatives" (Kirkpatrick 2009). Hospitals benefited from their own special arrangement. After agreeing to $155 billion in health care savings under Medicare over a 10-year period, leading hospital associations gained an exemption from other kinds of future cost-cutting (Chaddock 2009). Insurers got most of all. By agreeing not to oppose a ban on the practice of excluding applicants with pre-existing conditions, the industry received the president's endorsement of the individual mandate and, by extension, millions of new paying customers. Despite this understanding, insurers fought hard to shape legislation, contributing between $10–20 million toward attack ads against reform bills moving through Congress (Stone 2010). They were not alone in committing to this expensive strategy. According to the public interest group Common Cause, major health care interests spent roughly $1.4 million per day lobbying Congress when consideration of health reform was in full swing (Zaharoff 2009).

Voters always loomed in the background as the ultimate audience Democrats and Republicans wanted to persuade when trading arguments about reform. The public was well aware of cost and access problems in the U.S. health system, and it strongly backed reform in general. A month after Obama launched his health reform initiative, 59 percent of Americans agreed reforming health care "is more important than ever" (Kaiser Health Tracking Poll 2009). But the Administration needed to win over Americans to its particular brand of reform. Obama took to the stump and airwaves with a series of speeches, town hall forums, and primetime news conferences, all to communicate his plan directly to the people. The White House even launched a webpage, "Health Insurance Reform: Reality Check," as a way of clearly outlining the initiative. Results were frustratingly mixed. A February 2010 poll showed most Americans were against "Obama's health care reform plan," but, paradoxically, a majority supported specific provisions included in the bill (Kliff 2010). Certainly, the president would have liked to claim public opinion was behind him as political leverage in dealing with opponents, but never could he do this convincingly.

Institutional workings of the U.S. Congress also made reform difficult. Worried about opposition forces gaining traction, the Administration urged lawmakers to move quickly. Congress is designed to be a slow moving body, however (Peterson 2008). The Senate Finance Committee alone deliberated over health reform for months in a failed attempt to find common ground between the two parties. Soon, the 2009 summer recess was at hand. Upon returning home to their home districts, Congressional members found themselves in the midst of explosive town hall meetings, where for weeks on end an outpouring of citizen protests played on national television. Opponents stoked public unease using symbolic language to strike at deep-seated fears over **"socialized medicine,"** **rationing**, and an out-of-control federal government.

The politics of health reform also showed just how difficult it is to get a bill through a body like Congress without overwhelming majority support. Democrats controlled both houses of Congress, but not with a reliable veto-proof margin. After Massachusetts Senator Ted Kennedy died in August of 2009, he was replaced by Republican Scott Brown the following January. This meant Democrats lost their "super majority" of 60 seats, increasing the possibility of **filibustering** by the opposing party—a practice that has become easier and more common due to changes in institutional rules and procedures over the years. Republicans marched in lockstep, giving virtually no votes to reform throughout the months when legislation worked its way from committee to floor in both chambers. Competition and dissent in the Democratic Party complicated the Administration's task. House Democrats finally passed a bill substantially different from the more conservative Senate measure. Additionally, in the waning days of debate, a right-to-life faction within the Democratic Party withheld support from any legislation that did not de-link federal dollars from funding for abortive services (MacGillis 2010).

So, in the end, the president did not get all he wanted, not least a public option forcing private insurers to compete with a government plan. It is perhaps remarkable Obama and the Democratic leadership got as much as they did from this tumultuous policy episode. The rocky ride will continue as the nation moves forward into implementation and future revisions to the ACA gain consideration. A comparative perspective may prove useful in broadening our reflections on the politics of health reform.

After the Big Bang

Policy analysts mark an important distinction between legislation that takes incremental steps and legislation that accomplishes true innovation. An **incremental policy** brings about relatively small adjustments in the status quo, such as modest expansion of an existing program, while an innovation is associated with a marked shift in philosophy, level of resource allocation, or program mechanism within a policy area. Sometimes policy innovations have been termed **"big bang"** policy making. A major overhaul of this type promises much and risks much simultaneously.

While the Affordable Care Act did not go as far as many health reformers would have liked—for example, it did not try to upend the employment-based insurance system—the law qualifies as one of the biggest breakthroughs in the history of U.S. health policy. According to the *New York Times*, it represents "the most expansive social legislation enacted in decades" (Stolberg and Pear 2010). The political system has now reverted to more standard incrementalist mode. We are not likely to deviate from this path any time soon. Critics sometimes bemoan the limitations of a process that creeps forward by small steps and narrow fixes. But what does the experience of other nations tell us about the interplay between incrementalism and big bang policy making in the ongoing evolution of health reform?

France can be seen as a "poster child" for the promising possibilities of incrementalism (Rodwin 2003). Created in 1928, public health insurance in the "Hexagon" country initially covered only a segment of lower-wage workers. From this modest beginning, the system developed. In 1945, policy makers expanded the program to encompass all industrial and commercial workers and their families. In 1961 and 1966, farmers and agricultural workers and independent professionals, respectively, were brought into the fold. In 1974, the French government finally declared insurance protection should be universal, although the final 1 percent of the population did not gain comprehensive coverage until 2000. In this same year, the World Health Organization issued a report ranking the French National Health Insurance system best in the world.

Why did the French take so long to achieve universal coverage? How did they do it? Today the French government operates under a "strong state" model with considerable capability for bypassing recalcitrant interests in the policy process (Wilsford 1991). This has not always been the case. Prior to constitutional changes, industry groups in the health sector were able to block comprehensive reform by exploiting veto points within the French parliament. Following establishment of the Fifth Republic in 1958, the French president acquired power to issue legislation directly through decree or ordinance, and to put legislation before the people in referendum form (Immergut 1992). Although the U.S. president is unlikely to gain such authority, the French example illustrates that incremental reforms, however they are achieved, can add up over time. As health policy scholar Victor Rodwin (2003) points out, "the evolution of French NHI demonstrates that it is possible to achieve universal coverage without a 'big bang' reform." Instead, Rodwin suggests the U.S. "accept piecemeal efforts that extend social insurance coverage to categorical groups beyond current beneficiaries of public programs" (p. 36).

On the other hand, a British reform episode warns of the backlash that dramatic policy change can provoke. In 1991, Margaret Thatcher's government pursued a system-wide big bang reform "disdaining consensus, experiment, and incrementalism and overriding strident opposition from the medical profession and others" (Klein 1995: 300). The design of Thatcher's competition initiative will be detailed in the next chapter, but a political observation belongs here. In running roughshod over providers, especially physicians, the Thatcher administration revealed what Rudolph Klein describes as "one of the central paradoxes of health care reform" (p. 319). Enacting reform upsets groups within the existing system whose support is critical to the very success of policy change. Thus, as physician dissatisfaction spread to patients and the British public at large, a political gain for the Thatcher administration soon turned into a liability.

In health policy making there are times of incrementalism and times of comprehensive change, and reformers need to do what they can with the former while awaiting the latter. This is a true statement, as far as it goes, but an oversimplified depiction of the situation, as scholars like Columbia University's Lawrence Brown (2005) have discussed. The politics of incrementalism may actually feed the formation of narrow constituencies contributing little to big bang reform. The notion of a dichotomy between policy incrementalism and policy innovation itself could distract reformers from accurately surveying the political landscape. Among other possibilities, attention must be given to *large* incremental steps as well as *small* innovations—Brown prefers the concept of "moderate-sized political explosions"—in setting the policy agenda within an imperfectly reformed U.S. health care system.

Ideology versus Problem Solving

As President Obama prepared his health care address to Congress in fall of 2009, the *LA Times* concluded his "main task must be to retrieve the issue from the clutches of **ideology** and restore the search for ideas to the forefront" (Hiltzik 2009). Today, a nascent effort has sprouted forth in the United States to encourage just this kind of shift from the politics of ideology to a politics of problem solving.

In late 2010, a coalition of Democrats, Republicans, and Independents committed to promoting civil discourse and bipartisan solutions launched the No Labels movement. According to William Galston, senior fellow at the Brookings Institution and one of the group's co-founders, "The No Labels point is that there are a whole lot of people in this country outside of Washington who are more interested in solving problems than scoring points" (NPR 2011). Some prominent leaders agree. When Senator Evan Bayh, an Indiana Democrat, recently announced he would not be seeking a third term in office, this was his stated reason: "There is much too much partisanship and not enough progress. Too much narrow ideology and not enough practical problem solving" (Becker and Zeleny 2010).

Anyone questioning the desire to tame the passions and polemics of the U.S. health care debate may want to hear about the country–continent of Australia. Australia shares with the United States "a history of intense and ongoing controversy surrounding health care" (Gray 1996: 588). As a parliamentary democracy, however, the majority party in Australia can marshal votes for its legislative program much more effectively than under the fitful U.S. system. Deep ideological divisions combined with an institutional setting conducive to change have led national health policy in Australia to "oscillate" between starkly opposing policy solutions.

In 1972, the Labor Party established Medibank as the nation's first compulsory health insurance plan. Then, before Medibank could be fully implemented, Malcolm Fraser's Liberal-National Coalition government took office and began its dismantlement. By 1981, free hospital care had been abolished and a private health insurance scheme reinstated. Two years later, the Labor Party returned to power and re-established national health insurance, this time under the moniker of "Medicare." During the economic recession of the early 1990s, private hospitals, private health funds, and physicians seized the moment to spearhead a national debate (ultimately unsuccessful) over "reprivatization," or the reduction of Medicare to a welfare program with everyone else in the country forced to buy private insurance (Gray 1996).

According to Australian policy scholar Gwendolyn Gray (1996), this ideological push-and-pull forced important health concerns about the shape of the delivery system and the role of prevention and primary care off the table in this period. Policy makers were simply too busy debating the unsettled philosophical question of "public versus private" to grapple with lesser problems of a more functional nature. The conflict of "irreconcilable ideologies" continued at strength into the 21st century (Gray 2004).

America is not Australia, but it is hard not to think of current legal and fiscal maneuvering within the U.S. to cancel the 2010 reform before it can even get off the ground. One also notes with concern how pragmatic matters, such as the application of **evidence-based medicine** to control the costs of care, are growing more and more politicized after being drawn into the unstable orbit of our national reform debate (Gerber and Patshnik 2010).

How does a country move beyond ideology once accustomed to the high-octane exchange of emotive symbols and inflammatory rhetoric? It is a troubling quandary that will not be easily disposed of here. Less clamorous dogma, more sober attention to planning, management, and monitoring of results—this is hardly a rousing call to arms, but it just may be the right prescription for rebalancing the political discourse surrounding health care in America.

Dealing with Special Interests

Hospitals, insurers, drug manufacturers, and physicians influenced the content of the Affordable Care Act in lasting ways. Needless to say, officials will face continued demands from these and other health care interest groups as the reform program moves forward. No simple recipe exists for dealing with special interests in the policy process, crucial though this may be for effective government action. As Constance Nathanson (2005) has commented, "In the United States, we are subject to periodic debates about the legitimacy of interest-group politics. This form of political representation is, nevertheless, well established in our system of government and is unlikely to disappear, however much hand wringing it generates …" (p. 195). It may help, nonetheless, to complement our nation's own story of health reform with an awareness of stakeholder challenges in other health systems.

Development of national health insurance in Israel illustrates how a reform of health *policy* may actually precipitate a corresponding reform of health *politics* (Chinitz 1995). For many years, a tri-part alliance of interests dominated Israel's health policy arena. The three groups included the nation's largest sickness fund, Kupat Cholim Clalit (KHC), the General Federation of Labor (GFL), and the national Labor Party. Membership in the KHC was contingent on membership in the GFL, a fee to join both organizations inextricably linking the two. This association, strengthened by cooperation from the Labor Party, created a powerful "subsystem" capable of blocking policies antithetical to the interests of KHC.

During the late 1980s, however, growing public dissatisfaction with the health care system, labor unrest, and financial instability at KHC led to a State Commission of Inquiry. Also during this time, a younger generation of Labor Party members began to openly oppose the tri-part relationship described above. Their resistance stemmed mainly from growing consumer dissatisfaction with the KHC and its inability to match the services provided by other sickness funds. Many members with means exited from the KHC and GFL, which, in turn, weakened the GFL's political power. Following elections in 1992, Haim Ramon, a prominent member of Labor's younger generation and opponent of the KHC–GFL link, stepped into the position of health minister. Ramon, along with other prominent Labor Party leaders, endorsed the commission's recommendation for a national health insurance program separating the GFL and KHC (Twaddle 2002).

New legislation, enacted in 1995, established universal coverage in Israel by requiring all residents to choose among four sickness funds, one of them the KHC. The Ministry of Health became responsible for defining population benefits while gaining a pre-eminent role in health care planning and budgeting. Further, primary funding for insurance coverage would now flow through the tax system, to be allocated to sickness funds by the National Health Insurance Institute (Okma et al. 2010). In this way the KHC lost much of its decision-making influence within Israeli health policy. As David Chinitz (1995) puts it, this was a reform establishing not just a new set of policies, but a new political power structure as well: "In Israel, the venue of health policy has shifted, with influence moving from the sickness funds to actors and institutions that previously played a lesser role in health policy or that are being newly created" (p. 926).

For an American audience, this tale seems a timely reminder of the fluidity of power politics as well as reform's potential impact in re-setting the table of players for the next round of policy decisions. Under the ACA, our country will be inventing or transforming a host of government agencies, legislative committees, cost-cutting commissions, state-based insurance exchanges, and other entities. The health system will operate differently because of these institutional changes and so, too, will the politics of health care. New obstacles, opportunities, and venues of interaction all will surface in the relationship between government and mobilized interests.

The Netherlands presents another kind of experience with special interests. The tradition of **neocorporatism** in Dutch health care, also known as the "Polder model," emphasizes stakeholder representation while giving veto power to powerful groups claiming they will be impacted adversely by a policy proposal. Although this consensus-based practice has translated into substantial stability within Dutch politics, it also tended to retard, or even derail, new directions in health policy. During the 1990s, the Dutch Parliament drastically reduced stakeholder participation in public policy decisions. As a result, the government was able to pass a significant health reform in 2006, one based on a proposal strikingly similar to those stymied in earlier years (Okma and De Roo 2009). This is but a brief rendering of a much more complicated story. Suffice it to say, however, that the situation suggests an insight worth generalizing: While working cooperatively with interest groups may be effective to a point, there comes a time when meaningful change can require government officials to muster the courage to act independently.

The Outside Game of Politics

In the politics of policy making, there are "inside" and "outside" games. The inside game involves building support for proposals among lawmakers and organized stakeholders by such strategies as "logrolling" (trading favors), personal appeals, pressure from party leaders, and other forms of deal making and compromise (Peters 2004). The outside game is all about gaining public backing, typically through use of the media and other methods of mass communication. The outside game went badly for President Obama as he pursued health reform in 2009–2010. Although a concerted and serious effort, the Administration's PR campaign yielded uncertain results in the opinion polls and ultimately became overshadowed by a rancorous season of local protests. Events in other nations can shed light on this complex issue of public opinion formation and its role in health policy reform.

There are times and places when public opinion acts as a deciding factor in the health reform equation. In his comparative study of the creation of the British National Health Service (NHS) and U.S. Medicare program, Lawrence Jacobs (1993) asks why two countries so similar would adopt such different health reforms. He traces the answer to the emergence of formal opinion polling in both countries along with the growing sensitivity of lawmakers and other government officials to popular preferences. Jacobs argues that Britain's long history of government-provided health services fostered greater public openness to a state-administered, universal health care system. Americans had no such experience and were, as a result, only willing to support the more limited Medicare entity. Lawmakers' awareness of public opinion not only "loaded the dice" in favor of particular policy alternatives within each country, it also outweighed the opposition of prominent interest groups.

Yet the expressions of public opinion within health policy making are multiform around the globe. In 1992, after passing legislation to restructure the nation's health care financing, New Zealand officials were met with both a hostile press and disenchanted public (MacLeod 1994). Within just a few months, the government had to back off from implementing many provisions of its new law, and the incumbent party nearly suffered defeat the following election. In a curious sequence of events in Italy, a groundswell of public support for a questionable cancer cure compelled the government to take a significant chunk out of the small budget allotted for medical research to confirm the treatment's inefficacy (Benelli 2003). In recent decades, pressure to expand private health care funding within Canada's public system has fanned the flames of controversy. In this case, public opinion results have been used to gauge public preferences, frame policy options, and sway the outcome of debate (Contandriopoulos and Bilodeau 2009).

In all democratic societies, then, public opinion is a phantom giant, virtually irresistible when awakened but often bemused and subject to manipulation. Evidence speaks clearly to the need for leaders to converse more effectively with the citizenry by providing information, clarifying options, and explaining the relative costs and benefits of action versus inaction whenever important health policy decisions must be made. A system responsive to the voice of the people may be a founding ideal of American government, but the challenge is perennial and no less perplexing today than it ever was.

Health Reform and the Politics of Budgetary Shortfall

Anticipating the future in politics is always looking through a glass darkly. When it comes to health care, however, one fact seems plain, and that is the growing linkage between policy choices and dire budgetary conditions.

A clear sign of the times came in April of 2011 when Republican Paul Ryan, chairman of the House Budget Committee, proposed a plan for the 2012 federal budget cutting spending by $5.8 trillion over the next decade. Central to Ryan's vision is a dramatic retooling of Medicare, which the lawmaker has described as heading down "an unsustainable path" made even less viable by the Affordable Care Act. Rather than maintain the existing public entitlement, Ryan would convert Medicare into a voucher program by giving seniors fixed sums to help them buy coverage on the private market (Hulse and Calmes 2011). While many fellow Republicans pulled away from this initiative as unrealistic, it signaled an impulse for fundamental restructuring of U.S. health policy born of the collision between deficit reduction and entitlement reform as national issues. No mere budgetary adjustment, such a shift toward privatization threatened the principle of comprehensive affordable coverage established for the elderly over the last half century.

The economic downturn of the past few years has given rise to health cuts on the international scene as well, challenging nations across Western Europe and elsewhere to find ways to maintain their universal coverage systems in the face of acute fiscal shortfalls. France saw vigorous public protests over the government's adoption of increased cost sharing combined with reductions in health services (Gauthier-Villars 2009). Large demonstrations against cuts in social programs, including health care, have also taken place in Spain and Portugal. The response to **austerity measures** varies depending on culture and the configuration of political forces within different countries. Still, the theme of the day in health policy on all sides is the search for new efficiencies due to seismic shifts in public financing. Recognizing the impact of budgetary duress on health systems as a global phenomenon, the World Health Organization issued a public statement in April of 2009 calling for a cooperative effort among nations to yield "systems that are stronger, more efficient and more equitable than those that are currently under such serious threat" (Chan 2009).

Little precedent exists for such coordinated international strategizing in health policy. However, there *is* substantial past experience with retrenchment at home and abroad to outline possible future patterns. In the U.S. as elsewhere around the world, coming years are likely to bring forth health care proposals ranging from across-the-board cuts, to radical policy deconstruction (from the right and the left), to repair of existing policy frameworks. "Dedistribution" may produce conflict and deadlock, on the one hand, but it can also stimulate extraordinary political formations focused on resolving chronic policy contradictions, on the other (Light 1995; Rogne et al. 2009). (A telling case in point is the momentous fight over the U.S. debt and deficit.) The critical questions are: How much of a crisis will be necessary to jumpstart this political project? And how creatively will leaders respond after all recognize what is at risk?

Conclusion

We inhabit an era of intense partisan strife packaged and purveyed under the glare of round-the-clock cable television. Political drama is part of everyday life, so much so that a "quiet news day" may seem abnormal, the worrying calm before another major public storm. It's enough to make even the most seasoned political veteran fatigued at times. A few weeks before passage of the Affordable Care Act, in February of 2010, President Obama commented to CBS reporter Katie Couric: "I would have loved nothing better than to simply come up with some very elegant, academically-approved approach to health care [that] didn't have any kinds of legislative fingerprints on it and just go ahead and have that passed. But that's not how it works in our democracy" (Farber 2010). Nor is it how things work in other countries either. Institutional and cultural factors yield a fascinating tableau of health reform experiences and outcomes around the world. From this cross-national perspective comes an atlas of political probabilities inviting to consult in the aftermath of U.S. health care reform.

DISCUSSION QUESTIONS

1. In what ways did political factors shape the Affordable Care Act? How did the values and interests of different groups come to be represented in the process of health reform?
2. How would you rate the Affordable Care Act as a response to the problems of the U.S. health system?
3. Based on the national experiences outlined in this chapter, what advantages and disadvantages do different systems of government possess for policy making in an area like health care?
4. Which international trends in the politics of health reform seem most relevant for the U.S. over the coming decade?

V: Health Policy Design

Wisdom favors public policies characterized by simple design and clear cause–effect relationships. Such straightforwardness has often been missing from U.S. health reform efforts due to competing policy goals, a political environment populated with influential interests, and the tendency for law making to become ensnared in value-laden ideological debates. The promise of comparative analysis lies in the pragmatic opportunity to compile examples of policy interventions elsewhere whose intellectual rationale and operational history are well documented and whose positive outcomes justify serious scrutiny. Herein lies a wellspring for ongoing innovation in health policy development, if only Americans would be sufficiently curious and open-minded. When it comes to national problem solving, there is nothing ignoble about "systematically pinching ideas," especially if it offers a prudent way to combine art and science, invention and selection, in public policy design (Schneider and Ingram 1988).

Government's Toolbox

"There oughta be a law against that!" This colloquialism expresses the sentiment—part outrage and part desperate plea—that government must control intolerable behavior in society. "There oughta be a program for that!" This second cry is complementary and likely to be heard from those who desire government to fill some gap, or correct a maldistribution, in the private provision of resources.

In a nation like the United States that prizes limited government and personal liberty, both are reluctant statements—until a problem hits close to home. Then the appeal to government is reflexive, whether it's from out-of-work individuals calling for extended unemployment benefits, homeowners wanting help with outsized mortgage payments, or automakers and Wall Street bankers angling for enormous public bailouts. Suddenly the notion of government sitting passively on the sidelines becomes anathema. Time has come to render the world a saner, safer, and more predictable place, and it is government's job to make it happen.

Even when pressure rises irresistibly for government to step in and fix a social problem, what should be done and how? Often the answer is unclear. Should there be a rule or prohibition enforced under threat of legal sanction? Or does a more subtle approach fit the circumstances, perhaps financial incentives and other inducements to realign the status quo? Maybe this is the moment for government to enter boldly into a new domain of activity, competing with private actors to produce greater efficiency or accepting responsibility for a function or population group shunned by the market place? In reality, government officials have a toolbox filled with many options (Bardach 2009).

States learn a lot from each other's public policies, both those that succeed and those that fail. The federal government learns a lot from the states, particularly when numbers of them commit to the same policy and test it under different circumstances over time. When we talk about learning lessons from abroad, it represents another form of opportunistic fact gathering to inform policy design here at home. Other nations can offer valuable policy examples outside the range of U.S. experience, although an example that seems *too* foreign runs the risk of being readily dismissed. Nonetheless, increasing competitiveness and sociopolitical connection globally is a fact of life that requires all countries to monitor policies and practices in an international context.

The tricky thing is that selection of tools in policy design is not just about what works best, even if that were crystal clear to all observers. Politics enters in as powerful groups fight against government proposals infringing on their interests. There is also the cultural dimension discussed in Chapter II. In the consideration of ends and means in policy development, pressure is great for strategies that hew closely to popular expectations concerning use of public authority.

This discussion has direct relevance for health reform in the United States. Recognizing the prevalence of problems in this sector—gaps in insurance coverage, soaring costs, devastating impacts on individuals, families, businesses, and government itself—has not been difficult. Indeed, the problems appear all around us in a way impossible to ignore. But which instruments hold promise of offering the optimum policy solution?

The Affordable Care Act represents one response to this question, its complicated content drawing on multiple policy tools simultaneously. New regulatory penalties, taxes, government subsidies, government management, and reliance on private market mechanisms are all blended in a complex recipe inspired by the patchwork of existing U.S. health policy.

But this law is also a work in progress. This fact is evident in provisions for ongoing fact-finding plus demonstration programs on coverage expansion, cost control, quality improvement, preventive medicine, and other items. These, of course, are much the same issues with which health policy makers in other countries have been struggling for decades.

Coverage in the Balance

Earlier it was noted that foreigners often mistake health care in the United States to be a strictly private system. Conversely, many Americans typecast the health systems of other countries, particularly European nations, as all big government programs. In fact, a surprising diversity surfaces when one looks at how health insurance coverage is provided abroad.

Two policy design options dominate the universal health plans of economically advanced nations (Carrin and James 2005). The first is financing through government taxation, including general income taxes on individuals and businesses, local government taxes, and taxes specially earmarked for health care. The second is financing through **social insurance**, in which payroll-based contributions are collected from employers, employees, or both, for a statutory fund while government makes payments on behalf of those without means.

The health system of Canada, more than any other single country, has been examined—one really needs to say "argued about"—as a potential model for the United States. Canada presents a straightforward example of universal insurance through public financing (Health Canada 2011). Through personal and corporate taxes, sales taxes, payroll levies, and other revenue sources, Canada's federal, provincial, and territorial governments collect the funds. The 10 provinces play the lead role, while the federal government provides cash and tax transfers to lower levels of government consistent with guidelines from the Canada Health Act. In terms of the OECD's latest classification scheme, Canada has a "public contract model" in which private providers deliver the majority of services (Deber 2009). Most hospitals are non-profit entities; most physicians are in independent private practice. Canadian health care certainly has its controversies—waiting lists, fiscal strain, tension between federal and provincial authorities, and the emerging use of private insurance to give quicker access to services also covered under government's Medicare plan (Tuohy 2009). Still, population health indicators in Canada rank among the best in the world, and a solid base of popular support undergirds the universal public program (Soroka 2007).

This upside probably matters little for an American audience given how polarizing the Canadian **single-payer system**, and its identification with the specter of "socialized medicine," has become. Canada has "socialized financing" of medicine, an important distinction to make *vis à vis* countries where there is outright public ownership of health facilities and providers work for the government. As to how the Canadian model would actually perform in a country like the United States, which spends 90 percent more per capita on health care than its northern neighbor, one can only wonder. American single-payer die-hards continue the fight where and how they can. "Medicare for All" proposals are regularly reintroduced in Congress. Vermont and California are now reviewing bills combining universal coverage and single-payer principles with an eye toward qualifying for "state innovation" waivers under the Affordable Care Act's Section 1332. So far, however, there is little to contradict the judgment of health insurance expert William Glaser (1993: 700) who stated nearly 20 years ago: "Whatever its merits, the Canadian health financing system will never be enacted in the United States."

Seemingly more relevant to America's current challenge of edging toward universal coverage is the social insurance approach (Jacobs and Goddard 2000). A common model in Western Europe, it can be found in the countries of Austria, Belgium, France, Germany, Luxembourg, and The Netherlands. Elsewhere in the world, Costa Rica, Israel, the Republic of Korea, and Japan all have social health insurance systems (Carrin and James 2005). Many countries in the developing world—Kenya, The Philippines, Vietnam, and India, among them—are likewise implementing versions of this same policy. As suggested by this listing, the social insurance model is compatible with a broad gamut of institutional and organizational arrangements concerning the number of funds through which coverage can be obtained, membership contributions, employers' financial responsibilities, scope of benefits, functions of private insurance, and government's administrative and regulatory role (Saltman, Busse, and Figueras 2004).

For a country like the U.S., where **pluralism** and choice are watchwords of the health sector, this flexible framework is arguably much more feasible than a full-blown system of public finance could ever be. Moreover, a typical pattern in social health insurance has been incrementalism. Most countries graduate to universality over time by dint of encompassing additional occupational categories, types of businesses, and population groups under public and private financing (Carrin and James 2005). The Affordable Care Act positions the U.S. nicely for heading down this well-worn path. Could the new state exchanges under ACA evolve from brokering entities into strong institutional structures for health insurance expansion and oversight in the mode of social health insurance? A homegrown American adaptation is not inconceivable, although the scale of change involved in such a transformation—programmatically and philosophically—should not be underestimated.

The German system is a noteworthy example of social health insurance, one recommended enthusiastically to U.S. health reformers by some policy scholars (Henke, Murray, and Ade 1994; Jackson 1997; Reinhardt 2009). Germany has hundreds of "sickness funds" organized on the basis of companies, regions, occupational groups, and guilds. Funds are private, non-profit entities that collect contributions, pool risk, and provide benefit packages under regulatory supervision by the federal government. Doctors in office-based ambulatory care tend to be private practitioners, while the hospital sector includes public, non-profit, and private facilities. Federal law mandates most categories of workers in the country join a sickness fund, the costs shared between employee and employer, but enrollees can make changes from one fund to another. Government contributes for those elderly, disabled, and unemployed. Self-employed individuals and others above a certain income level can either join a sickness fund or purchase private insurance. Praising the German way of health care, T. R. Reid (2009: 67) writes: "The package of benefits is generous ... The quality of care is world-class ... Germans spend less time waiting for care than Americans do ... Patients can choose any doctor or hospital, and insurance must pay the bill."

Of course, Germany and other European social health insurance systems possess one critical ingredient still absent from the U.S. context, namely, nationwide comprehensive coverage guaranteed under law. Obama's Affordable Care Act does not guarantee coverage; it merely moves the country in the direction of greater coverage. How fast will we progress toward goals of the bill (and beyond to universality)? The whole program is a giant math equation in which insurance outcomes, on one side, are a function of trends in employment-based coverage, expansion or contraction of state Medicaid programs, and the affordability of health plans offered through new health exchanges, on the other. Nor are coverage levels standardized outside the exchanges.

If the ultimate goal of health reform in the U.S. is universal coverage at a minimum level of adequacy—as many ACA supporters say it is—then the current design is a package of relatively weak instruments judged internationally. Still to be seen is where the balance between substance and symbolism will tilt as this federal bill becomes operating policy. Like some large public transit vehicle that needs brakes as well as steering to get where it is going, prospects are contingent on the stubborn task of cost control.

The Universal Bane of Costs

Rising health care costs are ubiquitous around the world, a problem for which no nation can yet claim a long-term solution. Each year the OECD publishes a careful accounting of health spending for its member nations. According to latest data for 2008, more than half this group now spends 8 percent or more of gross domestic product on health care (Kaiser Family Foundation 2011b). When health spending rises faster than overall economic growth, its share of GDP increases. This is exactly what has been happening over the past 50 years. Going back to 1960, no OECD country for which data are available spent more than 6 percent of GDP on health (Oxley and MacFarlan 1995). In 2008, only one country, Mexico, fell below 6 percent. All countries experienced marked increases in health expenditures per capita over the past several decades. Between 1980 and 2008, real annual growth rates (after correcting for inflation) have placed in the range of 2–4 percent.

So it is that the U.S. finds itself in good company when it comes to increasing health care costs. What is distinctive about the American situation, however, is how far out on the distribution we have strayed. On September 30, 2009, Mark Pearson, head of OECD's Health Division, submitted a statement to the U.S. Senate's Special Committee on Aging analyzing the health expenditure data collected by his organization (Pearson 2009). He made several memorable points highlighting the disparity between the U.S. and other countries. The U.S. spends more of its national income on health than anywhere else, despite the lack of universal insurance coverage. In 2007, health expenditures were 16 percent of GDP in the U.S., compared to 11 percent in

France, the next highest country. Even the U.S. government spends a greater amount on health care than do governments in other countries. In fact, among OECD members in 2007, only Norway and Luxembourg spent more per capita on health in public dollars than the United States. U.S. spending on administrative services within its health system is about twice the average of OECD countries. Going beyond Pearson's presentation, physician income is another area in which the U.S. is an international outlier, with American doctors making three times the OECD average (Bodenheimer 2005). The role of for-profit insurance companies and hospitals in U.S. health care also comes with a high price tag due to the exceptionally high salaries paid to executives in some of these companies.

Public policies to contain health care costs can be categorized in various ways: supply-side versus demand-side strategies (Rapoport, Jonsson, and Jacobs 2009); budget setting, budget shifting, and direct and indirect regulatory controls (Mossialos and Le Grand 1999); and cost controls versus rationing (Blank and Burau 2010). However one dissects this subject, a principal theme dividing the U.S. and other countries is concentration of buying power.

The More you Buy, the More you Save

A "**monopsony**" is an economic market in which buyers, not suppliers, dominate. As developed nations around the globe have confronted rising health costs, the primary response has been to foster conditions of monopsony by strengthening the position of buyers through centralization, coordination, and consolidation. Stated in political terms, in the perennial struggle for societal resources, the use of public policy to concentrate health care buying power is a strategy for advantaging public over private interests (Marmor 1994). When buyers gain control of the payment process, it becomes a powerful tool for bargaining over prices, spending limits, and overall development of the system. By contrast, in the United States "a large and fluctuating group of private insurers, competing in a private marketplace, cannot be coordinated to manage the system as a whole" (Evans 2008: 447).

Canada concentrates buying power through public financing of health care and direct government administration of spending (Marmor and Mashaw 1994). Government is virtually the sole payer for services under the universal health insurance plan. Acting under this authority, provincial officials set fee schedules for physician services. Hospitals must operate with global budgets determined by government that specify a fixed amount of funding per year.

While Germany does not have a single-payer health system of this kind, it, too, has implemented a policy concentrating buying power. The national government limits spending by sickness funds in line with income growth in the country. There are regional fixed budgets for ambulatory care, and regional target volumes for pharmaceuticals. The sickness funds, in turn, negotiate prices and fees with providers, including global budgeting for hospital care (Wörz and Busse 2009).

More than 5,000 miles to the east lies the nation of Japan, whose culture and politics could not be more different from Germany's in most ways. Yet the Japanese health system relies on methods of cost control following a logic familiar to German policy makers (Ikegami 1991; Hisashige 2009). Japan's social health insurance system has three categories of plans: employment-based insurance, national health insurance, and a program of coverage for the elderly. Most providers are in the private sector. The Japanese government sets a nationally uniform fee schedule covering all procedures and products, including drugs. This schedule must conform to a government budget ceiling for health care based on Japan's GDP. Insurers and providers are important stakeholders in the negotiation process over these figures and rates, but government has greatest leverage of all.

Attempting to assess the effectiveness of single-payer versus all-payer cost containment internationally, researchers have arrived at mixed findings (see, e.g., Glied 2009). Should the cost-control function be carried out nationally or regionally? By public bureaucracies, or private bodies with delegated public authority? As Marmor and Mashaw (1994) have written, it appears to be "the *concentration* of financial responsibility, not its precise location, that is crucial to countervailing inflationary health pressures" (p. 82, emphasis in original). In addition, whatever the institutional backdrop, "[t]he political will to restrain health care costs is itself a necessary ingredient for success" (p. 83). As the U.S. pursues its own malleable reform, both insights merit attention.

Markets + Competition = More Regulation

Promotion of **competition** within health care markets is a policy design strategy aimed at reshaping supply *and* demand. Within American politics, increased competition has been a popular theme among those opposed to a larger government role in health care going back to the Reagan presidency. It was also a main component of President Clinton's proposed reform in the early 1990s. Small surprise, then, that our 2010 reform incorporates elements of competition alongside mandates, subsidies, and system controls. The emphasis on competition is hardly an isolated American development. Over the past two decades, other countries have also taken steps to introduce competitive incentives and pressures in the way they deliver and pay for health care.

One form taken by these experiments is the creation of quasi-markets for providers in countries with national health services or single-payer systems (Docteur and Oxley 2003). Great Britain presents an example of keen interest for the U.S. not only because of close bonds between our two countries, but also because American experts helped advise the changes. The British NHS was established shortly after World War II. It provides universal coverage paid for chiefly through general taxation. Great Britain has undergone two waves of competitive reforms (Brereton and Vasoodaven 2010). The first came under conservative Margaret Thatcher in the mid-1990s and focused on separating purchaser and provider functions within the government. This meant encouraging general practitioners (GPs) to take control of budgets for purchasing elective hospital services for their patients, while Health Authorities at the regional level bought other forms of care. Hospitals also became organized as "trusts" competing for patients from GPs and the authorities. Impacts of this policy shift were not easy to pin down subsequently in regard to quality or cost, and equity issues surfaced between patients served by fundholding and non-fundholding GPs (Le Grand 2007).

When Tony Blair's Labour government took office in 1997, it undid most of this initiative. Blair's own competitive approach eventually proved more complicated, but critical features included demand-side changes (formation of new purchasing entities on the community and regional levels) as well as supply-side changes (an expanded role for private and voluntary providers within the NHS). Patients gained more freedom of choice when accessing elective care services. Still a work in progress, the Blair policy is already under revision by a new British government, and implementation difficulties have occurred in several areas. One careful review of research on Britain's two waves of internal market restructuring concludes: "[T]he reforms have not been proven to bring about the beneficial outcomes that classical economic theory predicts of markets, including provider responsiveness to patients and purchasers; large-scale cost reduction; and innovation in service provision" (Brereton and Vasoodaven 2010: 10).

Another kind of pro-competition policy is seen in countries with multiple insurers, such as Belgium, the Czech Republic, The Netherlands, and Germany (Docteur and Oxley 2003). An interesting case with a long history of private insurance markets is Switzerland, which came briefly into the spotlight during the recent U.S. health reform debate. Switzerland has an individual mandate requiring all residents to purchase a health plan from a private nonprofit insurer, but the government subsidizes lower-income individuals to keep costs beneath a fixed percentage of income (Jacobs and Goddard 2000). Insurers, for their part, compete to attract customers on the basis of product benefits and costs. Regulation plays a big part in structuring how this works, beyond the compulsory health insurance requirement. Public authorities supervise insurance companies with respect to administration, accounting, and determination of premiums. The government also cross-subsidizes insurers so that high-risk subscribers do not get left by the wayside.

Often, the topic of health care competition is framed as a false choice between market and government. The promised benefits of increased competition among providers and insurers are substantial—if not always easy to document—but there are risks. Government has an important role in guarding against the latter by deciding "rules of the game" and by monitoring competitive behaviors. The Affordable Care Act encourages competition in several arenas, for instance, the formation of new Accountable

Care Organizations to integrate care for elders, and the functioning of new insurance exchanges as competitive marketplaces for affordable coverage. As these design structures take shape, the foreign lesson seems clear: "Reform experience in Europe has shown that the greater the reliance on market mechanisms, the greater the need for a reinvigorated state role" (Saltman and Figueras 1998: 101–102; see, also, Freeman 1998).

Cost Shifting through Cost Sharing

In 1980, Princeton health economist Uwe Reinhardt reported the reluctance of other nations to embrace **cost sharing** in health care. He linked this aversion to a commitment to progressive principles. That commitment has not withstood the test of time and budgetary scarcity.

A study of 18 European countries in the late 1990s found cost sharing to be a spreading policy that transcended tax-based and social health insurance methods of health system financing (Ros, Groenewegen, and Delnoij 2000). Cost sharing provisions included coinsurance (payment of a fixed percentage of charges), copayments (payment of a flat fee per episode of service), and/or deductibles (payment of a specified amount out-of-pocket before insurance coverage begins). By 2009, all OECD nations had in place cost sharing for prescription drugs, and only Spain, Canada, Denmark, and Great Britain did not have cost sharing for at least certain forms of publicly funded health care (Skinner and Rovere 2010).

National particulars are important for appreciating how cost sharing can be flexed as an ingredient of policy design. In 2009, the Kaiser Family Fund focused on cost sharing in three countries (Kaiser Family Foundation 2009). Germany and France have various coinsurance and copay requirements for hospital care, physician services, and drugs. So, too, does Switzerland, in addition to a range of annual deductible amounts depending on the private health plan. Yet each of these countries has limited the impact of cost sharing by exemptions based on health status, defined categories of vulnerable persons, types of treatment and services, and income level. Germany and France also give residents the option of purchasing private supplemental insurance to cover costs not reimbursed under the public system. These practices recognize the danger, always present under cost sharing, that excessive out-of-pocket costs will cause sick individuals to delay or neglect necessary treatment leading to poor health outcomes.

The cost-sharing provisions of the Affordable Care Act are at once intricate and ambivalent as policy design. Consider these motley details. On one hand, the law limits out-of-pocket spending in plans offered by health exchanges; it gives subsidies to individuals and families based on income to reduce cost-sharing amounts; and it eliminates cost sharing for preventive services under Medicare, exchange plans, and new health plans offered outside an exchange. On the other hand, "grandfathered" individual and employer-sponsored plans do not have to meet national cost-sharing limits; the lowest-tier insurance plans on exchanges will feature very high deductibles; and Medicaid programs will not be required to have the same coverage of preventive services as Medicare. According to early research, consumers find themselves struggling with "deep-seated confusion and lack of confidence" when presented with information about health plan cost sharing under ACA (Quincy 2011). And who can blame them? Whether this legal hodgepodge can survive for long without revision is uncertain, but other countries have good guidance to offer in crafting a policy more complete and consistent.

Why Aren't We Talking More about Quality?

Improved quality has long stood alongside increased access and cost control in defining the triad of major health reform objectives for U.S. policymakers. As stated in federal health planning legislation of the mid-1970s, "The achievement of equal access to quality health care at reasonable cost is a priority of the Federal Government" (Public Law 93-641, Sec. 2[a][1] 1975).

The 2010 campaign for health reform did not address these three objectives in equal measure. Tracking political developments during summer of 2009, health care ethicist Daniel Callahan aptly registered his consternation in the *New England Journal of Medicine*: "Although everyone seems to agree that controlling health care costs is no less critical a need than improving access to health care, the evidence suggests that cost control is not being seriously confronted." And when the president delivered his national speech in September to signal the urgency for health reform, quality received barely a mention, other than Obama's fending off demagoguery that his plan would "set up panels of bureaucrats with the power to kill off senior citizens." Here was a shrewd political calculus. As with cost control, quality improvement is a policy activity that excites provider suspicion in a way coverage issues do not. In addition, the public consistently gives high grades to quality of health care in the U.S. system (Jones 2010).

Unfortunately, none of this means real quality problems do not exist in American medicine. An extensive body of research has documented overuse, underuse, and misuse of health services (Institute of Medicine 2001; Bodenheimer 2003). The consequence is counted in thousands of preventable deaths and injuries annually. A field of investigation known as "**small-area analysis**" reveals tremendous unexplained variation in common medical procedures from community to community around the country. If only the right treatment were given to the right patient at the right time, many analysts figure, not only would health care be better, but costs could be lowered as well.

The difficulty lies in translating studies that are *policy relevant* into a *relevant policy* supported by physicians and other providers (Morone 2008). The Affordable Care Act took a long-range view of quality improvement, calling for a "National Quality Strategy" subsequently released by the U.S. Department of Health and Human Services in March of 2011. This document is a "broad roadmap" that formulates aims and priorities, cites existing programs and services consistent with these generalities, highlights ACA components designed to enhance quality, and "promotes collaboration among stakeholders in the Nation's health system" to improve delivery of care (p. 17). It marks the latest phase in a long conversation about how we might maximize health care quality in this country, if only enough of the right individuals and organizations could be persuaded to make it a priority.

The essential point for policy makers and other quality advocates in the U.S. to remember is this is not a quest we need undertake alone. Enhanced health care quality now ranks as a top concern for research and planning groups across the globe. Perhaps most significant at this time, the OECD has launched a Health Care Quality Indicators project to "measure and compare the quality of health service provision" cross-nationally based on dozens of statistical measures in different areas of practice and programming. A related goal is sharing **best practices** from selected countries to advance health administration and policy development for all (Kelley 2007). Thus, the rising issue of health care quality is another compelling instance of **convergence** among national health systems. It also supplies a further illustration of why, when it comes to U.S. health policy design, isolationism is a luxury too extravagant to afford.

Conclusion

Each year tens of millions of Americans head abroad avidly employing their cameras, journals, and open eyes to capture impressions of life lived elsewhere. Once back home, the travelers reflect on and share this experience, perhaps even allowing it, as the expatriate novelist Henry Miller once said, to inspire them with "a new way of seeing things." Study of comparative health systems represents its own kind of intellectual tourism, one in which programs and values abroad can be absorbed for discussion as we contend with our most tenacious problems here at home. The information gathered may be positive guidance, negative lessons about alternatives to avoid, or something subtler to interpret. All such data can be building blocks in the creative process of health policy design.

DISCUSSION QUESTIONS

1. This chapter suggests that, of various approaches for instituting universal coverage, the social insurance model might best suit the United States. What do you think? Should the U.S. follow the example of other nations and work toward this goal? Why or why not?

2. Sometimes it is argued that universal coverage and cost control represent contradictory objectives in health policy making. What light does the experience of other nations shed on this issue?

3. What is it about a social good like health care that complicates reliance on the model of market competition? Does it seem counterintuitive to you that many nations have found it necessary to increase government regulation as part of their effort to expand competition?

4. Cost shifting is a tempting approach to containing costs in health care, but what are the drawbacks of this strategy?

VI: Making a Reformed System Work

Once the legislative struggle ends, a bill enters the statute book and the arduous part of the policy process is over. Provisions of the law are now as good as set in stone, making it a simple matter to establish programs, **regulations**, and services faithful to the intent of those who proposed the adopted measure.

NOT! Laws often fail in their application; even those that succeed can become badly distorted over time. Not only is the political fight between supporters and opponents prone to continue during policy implementation, organizational and inter-organizational dysfunctions may produce a mix of intended and unintended consequences. It is not uncommon for reasonable assumptions about the behavior of those affected by a law—individuals, groups, institutions—to prove faulty in practice. Sometimes administrative problems can be anticipated, sometimes they cannot. Laws not working well must be adjusted. For all these reasons, as policy specialist James Anderson writes, "Policy implementation is neither a routine nor very predictable process. Why some policies succeed and others fail remains a challenging puzzle" (Anderson 2003: 193).

The more ambitious, controversial, and complex a piece of legislation, the more likely it will be subject to implementation troubles. The Affordable Care Act scores high on all these attributes. In one of the first books about the Affordable Care Act after it was signed into law, two eminent political scientists struggled to narrow down future scenarios: "Almost every outcome remains possible: sudden reversal, protracted defeat, or long-term success" (Jacobs and Skocpol 2010: 147).

An Overview of ACA Implementation Issues

Broadly speaking, the Affordable Care Act faces a pair of implementation obstacles. One is political resistance to the law. The other is the administrative challenge of turning the law into an operational program.

On the national level, the U.S. House of Representatives, which is now under firm Republican control, has emerged as the hub of attempts to repeal President Obama's health reform. The day after his party scored big electoral gains in November of 2010, incoming House Speaker John Boehner pledged to undo the "monstrosity" of the Affordable Care Act. In January, the House did pass a measure "Repealing the Job-Killing Health Care Law Act." However, it ran into a brick wall in the Senate, where

Democrats comprise the majority. The greatest threat to health reform lies not in outright cancellation, but in legislative skirmishes blocking its funding. Under this scenario, the program's timetable of implementation could easily unravel (Aaron 2010).

The risk of dismantlement increases if Republicans manage to capture more political ground in 2012. A few more seats in the House would not do it, nor would a shift in the Senate, even one establishing Republican control, so long as President Obama remains in office to **veto** repeal legislation. But a two-thirds majority for Republicans in both houses, or capture of the Oval Office, and all bets are off. Admittedly, this is a speculative scenario. Still, ACA foes are laboring to make the upcoming election a referendum on the Democratic reform. A "Repeal Pledge" prepared by a conservative women's group seeks to persuade congressional candidates to sign the following commitment:

> I pledge, if elected, to vote for all bills which seek to REPEAL the health care bill, HR 3590, signed into law on March 23, 2010.
>
> To that end, I would now and will in the next Congress endorse and vote for all measures, including discharge petitions, leading to its defunding, deauthorization, and repeal.
>
> (OBAMACARE Repeal Pledge 2011)

Presidential candidates are being asked to promise to "promote and sign" these same reform-reversing measures. So far among Republican presidential hopefuls, only Newt Gingrich has affixed his name to the document.

If the U.S. House of Representatives represents the hub of the ACA repeal effort, state legislatures in many parts of the country are its spokes. According to the National Council of State Legislatures, laws to "limit, alter or oppose selected state or federal actions" in line with the 2010 law have been proposed in more than 40 states (Cauchi 2011). It is a real grab bag that runs the gamut from nonbinding resolutions exhorting overturn of the law to declarations of the ACA "null and void" on the state level. The movement is chiefly symbolic, more important for creating an unruly atmosphere surrounding ACA implementation than for asserting a viable claim of state exemption.

Legal challenges come at the Affordable Care Act from another direction and could prove more formidable in the long run (Goldman 2011). Asserting the necessity for bringing everyone sick and healthy into the insurance market, authors of the statute categorized the purchase of coverage as interstate commerce, an activity Congress has authority to regulate. So states Sec. 1501: "The individual responsibility requirement provided for in this section ... is commercial and economic in nature, and substantially affects interstate commerce." Opponents of the law claim this individual mandate interprets the powers of the Constitution's interstate commerce clause too broadly, or that it incorrectly defines the decision *not* to buy insurance as regulable. Another major strand in the legal assault on the ACA, pertinent to both the expansion of Medicaid and employers' coverage requirement, centers on state sovereignty under the **Tenth Amendment** (Hayes and Rosenbaum 2010).

Where will this legal struggle end? As T. R. Goldman (2011) writes, it is "unknown whether the Supreme Court will limit any potential ruling to the individual mandate or will address the constitutionality of the broader health care reform law. Clearly, if the high court were to rule that the individual mandate or the entire law were unconstitutional, the effects on implementation of major provisions of the Affordable Care Act would be enormous" (p. 5). This has all the makings of a political cliffhanger, except, that is, for the tortuously slow path of legal decision making in our society. (For scale, think the last three installments of the Harry Potter saga, minus the magic but with a few of the same costumes.) At the time of this writing, approximately 30 lawsuits against the Affordable Care Act are pending, and appeals courts in Ohio, Georgia, and Virginia have issued inconsistent rulings. The Supreme Court had shown no eagerness to get involved, but a request by the U.S. Justice Department for a ruling has suddenly accelerated the timetable. The highest court of the land is now expected to formulate an opinion on the law by June of 2012, although the scope of review remains highly uncertain (Liptak 2011).

The reluctance of many state actors to embrace the Affordable Care Act is a problem for more than political reasons. The states must shoulder the principal burden in administering, monitoring, and enforcing this legislation. Writing in the journal *Health Affairs*, state health policy experts Alan Weil and Raymond Scheppach (2010) identified "three core state functions" that must be executed under reform: (1) expansion of Medicaid, (2) regulation of the changing private insurance market, and (3) creation of new insurance exchanges.

While states possess great experience in delivering services and running health programs, not least among them Medicaid and Children's Health Insurance, the scope and novelty of what they are now being asked to do is arresting. States differ markedly in managerial capacity and commitment to social programs. One can expect this variation to condition responses to health reform. What is more, the Affordable Care Act calls for exceptional coordination between federal and state governments. These are unsettling concerns to keep in mind when gathering insights from health policy implementation abroad.

Federalism and Health Policy: A Comparative Perspective

Comparative scholars distinguish between ***unitary* political systems** that have "only one meaningful level of government above the local level" and ***federal* systems** with "one or two meaningful levels of government above the local level, and each level has its own institutionally defined policy-making responsibilities" (Adolino and Blake 2011: 67). This contrast between unitary and federal types is useful, although polities range considerably in the assignment of policy, funding, and administrative roles even within the two polar categories. Most nations have unitary structures. Federal systems, however, are generally more common in larger and more developed countries. Many Western democracies whose health care systems have attracted American interest, including Germany, Canada, Australia, and Switzerland, share in common with our country the institution of federalism.

Even countries familiar to the U.S. that have received a lot of coverage in our media, namely Canada, are much more complicated operationally than most Americans realize, with noteworthy variation across parts of the country as well as significant intergovernmental conflict. In their comparative study of health policy and federalism, Canadians Keith Banting and Stan Corbett (2002) explain: "[T]he structures of government ... make some outcomes easier than others, and therefore influence the capacity of political agents to act, their perceptions of realistic policy alternatives, their strategic options, and their preferences" (p. 4).

Two topics studied in-depth by scholars interested in the impact of "multi-level governance" on health care are access and cost. As Banting and Corbett (2002) summarize, regional differences under federalism undermine the goal of geographic equity, although this is a situation managed better by nations with universal health systems than the United States. Cost containment also appears to favor unitary systems due to fragmented public decision-making under federalism.

Australian federalism takes the form of power sharing between the Commonwealth and state and territorial governments (Hancock 2002). The respective roles of these two levels are far from well ordered or distinct. States and territories remain very dependent on financial transfers from the national level, but overlap and redundancy complicate the relationship between units of government. Health care is a main battleground for controversies in Australian federalism. One instrument used to sort out the intergovernmental puzzle is the Council of Australian Governments (COAG). An institutional innovation dating back to the early 1990s, the COAG provides an ongoing forum for review of funding and policy issues by national and sub-national leaders. The body has played a central part in reforms relating to public health services, strengthening of consumer-oriented programs, and changes in hospital payment practices.

Quite different from Australia are the circumstances of federalism in Belgium (de Cock 2002). For most of its history, Belgium functioned as a unitary state, but it has evolved into a federation over the past several decades. The reason was to recognize and empower, to some extent, the country's distinct cultural and linguistic communities. In addition to the federal parliament, there are also Flemish, Walloon, and Brussels legislatures in those respective regions. Unlike Australia, governmental powers in Belgium are precisely defined to affirm national pre-eminence while minimizing overlap between different levels. Thus, the health care sphere operates primarily under control of the national social security system. Even so, communities/regions have acquired important responsibilities in health education and preventive medicine, as well as in running nursing homes. A topic of fervent debate in Belgian health policy is the distribution of national resources and, especially, the equity of allocations among regions. The national government's approach to these issues aims at flexibility, a combination of objective policy analysis and political negotiation (Choudhry and Perrin 2007).

Health reform in the United States not only creates an opportunity for re-examining the practices of our federal system, it demands it. Under the Affordable Care Act, there are so many shared responsibilities between federal and state governments, so many points of intersection between state initiative and national oversight, outcomes depend on deft management of federalism dynamics. One implementation analysis concludes: "States will have enormous short-term and long-term needs for assistance as they grapple with federal health reform legislation. The current resources provided to organizations that have worked in different capacities with states are not sufficient to meet the likely demand, urgency, and scope of work of federal health reform" (Weil et al. 2009: 7).

Technical issues of intergovernmental administration and finance can, in fact, touch on essential questions of inclusion and fairness (Banting and Corbett 2002). Consider the establishment of new health insurance exchanges as devices for expanding access to affordable coverage. The ACA encourages independence in the way states determine benefit design, access to exchanges, and administrative structure, even to the point of allowing multiple exchanges in a single state or regional exchanges serving multiple states. Yet how will minimum standards of equity and efficiency be met? And how will performance of state models be documented and communicated throughout the intergovernmental network in the interest of administrative learning? Reflecting on questions like these, one can appreciate the efforts of other countries, like Australia, to install consultative bodies charged with building intelligence and cooperation across governmental units in policy reform.

Medicaid is the premier intergovernmental program within U.S. health policy. One potential eligibility issue now coming into view under ACA is the unstable movement of enrollments back and forth between Medicaid and the new insurance exchanges as a result of shifts in income and family composition of low-income families (Sommers and Rosenbaum 2011). Several policy options involving the rules and functioning of Medicaid could ameliorate this situation, although not without strategic collaboration between state and federal authorities.

A bigger problem could exist in regard to Medicaid's fiscal soundness at a time of declining state revenues, high unemployment, and mandatory expansion of Medicaid eligibility. True, the ACA provides federal support to assist states with the latter, but only on a temporary basis. A longer-term solution is indicated, one guided by re-appraisal of the amount and types of **intergovernmental transfers** taking place within Medicaid. This predicament parallels those being faced by other nations with federal systems.

It has been proposed that health reform in the United States may require "refiguring federalism," that resolving equity and performance inconsistencies from one part of the country to another necessitates a new "compact" between federal and state governments (Brown 2009). In a country fearful of government-driven change, it probably does not help to state the situation so bluntly, but the facts suggest it is true. Analysis of comparative federalism and its policy lessons can help inform this process.

Did Someone Say "Rationing"?

Angry, fearful charges that President Obama wished to pervert the U.S. health system by introducing rationing became a colorful, if mystifying, dimension of the public debate over health reform in 2009–10. The origin of this claim has sometimes been attributed to ex-Alaska Governor Sarah Palin, who penned an op-ed for the *Wall Street Journal* in September of 2009 sympathizing with "many of the sick and elderly [who] are concerned that the Democrats' proposals will ultimately lead to rationing of their health care by—dare I say it—death panels" (Palin 2009). In fact, this sensational observation issued from multiple sources of conservative punditry whose lineage reaches back to the campaign against President Clinton's health proposal in the early 1990s (Rutenberg and Calmes 2009). However started, the rhetorical power of the "death panels" theme was palpable. A spate of negative ads hammered home the message, which soon found its way onto placards and banners in local protests.

This episode was remarkable not just for the way rationing charges distorted the health reform proposal—in particular, its provisions for end-of-life counseling and payment reform under Medicare—but also for the facile presumption that rationing does not already exist within American medicine. An "unrationed" system would be one in which all people enjoy access to all desired, or recommended, services at times and places of their choosing. Certainly, this situation does not describe the delivery of health care in the United States. Rather, as Jonathan Cohn (2011) writes in *The New Republic*,

> Rationing is already a fixture of our health care system. It happens every time an insurer says no to a treatment. It happens every time a doctor or hospital recommends against a procedure because it doesn't seem worth the cost. And it happens every time somebody forgoes care because it's too expensive.

The prevalence of cost-related barriers to health care in the U.S. versus other countries is striking, as Cohn underscores. In an international survey by The Commonwealth Fund in 2008, more than half of American adults with chronic health conditions reported access problems with respect to medications, doctor visits, or medical testing and treatments during the previous two years (Schoen et al. 2008). No other nation in the study came close to this mark.

This does not mean other governments fail to limit access. Canada and Britain, for example, manage utilization, particularly elective procedures, by means of waiting lines, and there are budgetary caps for health care (Klein 2009). However "rational" this rationing procedure might be, it is a form of saying "not now" or sometimes "no" that does not make affected citizens happy. And sometimes the lines do grow intolerably long, or mistakes occur in prioritizing care. But on what basis can these imperfect arrangements, which at least attempt to tie care to clinical need, be judged inferior to rationing decisions left in the whimsical hands of the marketplace?

As the Affordable Care Act makes health care more accessible, administrative and clinical decision-making in the health system will, of necessity, evolve. Can rationing practices in the United States be rendered more visible, open to discussion, and subject to ethical review? Perhaps, although this promises to rank among the most sensitive issues of health reform implementation. The ACA is already under political attack from those who denounce the law's Independent Payment Advisory Board as a mechanism for return of the "death panels" (Tantaros 2011). In fact, as health economist and rationing expert Henry Aaron (2011) notes, although the board could help identify savings possibilities in Medicare over coming years, its recommendations do not apply outside this program. Nor is the board permitted to broach the subject of rationing under the 2010 health reform statute.

In their review of health care around the world, Blank and Burau (2010) describe the different rationing strategies found in different types of health systems. In national health services, overall budgetary constraints and resource limitation (medical facilities, equipment, and personnel) follow logically from government control of the health sector. Social insurance systems are more likely to exclude particular services from the list of reimbursable items when defining coverage. Great Britain is a country that has also promoted evidence-based medicine through its National Institute for Health and Clinical Excellence. Whatever the setting, rationing is inherently divisive as officials search for an acceptable balance between justice and efficiency, between the scope and sustainability of coverage.

Even as health reform permits the United States to begin to turn away from rationing-by-market, there are good reasons to conclude that, in view of our culture and politics, Americans will continue to favor the methods of implicit rationing. The latter refer to "discretionary decisions made by managers, professionals, and other health personnel" endeavoring to manage wisely the finite resources put at their disposal (Mechanic 1997: 84). The approach of countries, like Sweden and The Netherlands, that appointed high-level committees to formulate principles of rationing as national public policy is ill suited to the United States (Ham and Brommels 1994). Nonetheless, health reform does bring new energy to bear on the possibilities of medical decision-making that manages to be patient-centered, rather than rule-bound, while adhering to definable medical and social standards (Mechanic 1997). The U.S. need not copy any other nation's approach to setting limits, so long as it recognizes resource allocation as a universal task of health policy. Blank and Burau (2010) make the point concisely: "It is simply not possible to meet the needs of all citizens without compromising goals" (p. 119).

Insurance Regulation

Under the Affordable Care Act, state health insurance exchanges must be in place and running by 2014. If that sounds like a leisurely time frame, it is not. The U.S. Department of Health and Human Services plans to review and approve state exchange efforts in 2013. If a state is not ready by this time, federal authorities could choose to intervene. A key preliminary step for putting exchanges in place is the drafting and passage of complicated authorizing legislation on the state level. By late summer of 2011, only about 10 states had taken such action (Baker 2011).

By contrast, insurers have been anything but slow off the mark in mobilizing to shape the implementation of reform. Behaving as any good industry association should, America's Health Insurance Plans, together with other company lobbyists, has been pressuring regulators to write rules friendly to the financial interests, business operations, and political engagement of insurers (Pear 2010). This activity marks an almost seamless transition from previous efforts in opposition to the enactment of reform. Significantly, when the Department of Health and Human Services announced proposed rules in July of 2011 governing the creation of insurance exchanges, the agency conceded to demands that insurers be allowed to sit on the oversight boards, and it neglected to require states to negotiate with insurance companies over benefit packages and prices (Appleby and Weaver 2011). This is an unwelcome development for consumer groups, who wanted exchanges to use their market power to protect the uninsured (Mathews 2011).

Concludes the *Wall Street Journal*: "By leaving a lot of flexibility, the new Obama administration proposal sets the stage for battles within states over how powerful exchange regulators will be" (Mathews 2011). On the one hand, issues facing state officials in designing exchanges are myriad; on the other hand, examples of how to go about this work are limited. Timothy Stoltzfus Jost, a specialist in health insurance law at Washington and Lee University, has identified a lengthy list of concerns related to successful operation of insurance exchanges in matters of governance, selection of subscribers, employer relations, certification of health plans, promotion of competition among insurers, consumer protection, and more (Jost 2010). Massachusetts and Utah created their insurance exchanges before passage of the Affordable Care Act and can offer advice to other states based on this invaluable experience. However, vast differences separate these two models highlighting the range of choices that must be made in adapting such structures to preferences and capabilities across the country. How state insurance commissioners handle their role under reform promises to be a bellwether of policy and management trends on the subnational level. While all commissioners face certain minimum responsibilities under ACA, the law's flexible framework allows for broad discretion concerning the vigorousness of regulatory enforcement. Commissioners will also need to decide how much independence to stake out when pursuing the agenda of cost control with powerful industry actors (Jacobson 2011).

It may seem ironic to suggest American officials look abroad for help in regulating private insurers. More and more, however, this is a domain where other nations have practical experience. As Jost (2001) has written: "Excepting a handful of lingering hard-line Communist countries, private health insurance exists everywhere" (p. 429). In some countries, it provides only a minor supplement to public benefits, but there are other national systems featuring universal coverage, such as Australia and Chile, in which as much as 25–30 percent of the population are privately insured.

In the latter situation, regulation of the private insurance market tends to be far-reaching. Issues of concern are not so different from those in the United States, including coverage of high-risk individuals, curbing the rising costs of insurance with age, limiting administrative expenses, consumer protection, promoting fair competition, and encouraging cost-effective forms of care (see, e.g., Wasem and Greß 2009). This is not the place for detailed examination of measures adopted by different countries in pursuit of these goals. Suffice it to note their relevance to current discussions in the United States about insurance exchanges, not to mention the overarching dilemma of fashioning a public–private partnership in the implementation of health reform.

Bringing in the Public

The "democratic deficit" refers to the gap between citizens and the policy process in contemporary society (Esfandiari 2010). As opinion polls document, this is a problem keenly felt in many nations, and few areas of government matter more to the public than decisions affecting the provision of health care.

Implementation of health reform crystallizes this issue within the United States. New venues for public participation in health care planning are coming into being under federal law in the governance of health insurance exchanges. States are also soliciting public comment on exchange design as they grapple with specific regulatory possibilities. These mark real opportunities for citizen voices to be raised (and hopefully heard) within the policy process, albeit in a carefully circumscribed way.

Are there ways to engage citizens more fully in policy making and management? When the United States launched its ill-fated health system planning initiative in the 1970s, this was largely unexplored territory. It continues to be so today. Research bodies like the OECD (2001a) have mapped numerous methods in use cross-nationally, but little knowledge exists about how best to accommodate the technical, political, and cultural strains associated with such a venture in practical democracy.

In general, comparative analysis shows more information about government is available to citizens globally than ever before (OECD 2001b). Public consultation on policy proposals is also on the rise. With respect to including citizens as partners in the policy process, however, examples are rare. One bright patch is the vast improvement in information and communication technologies not available to health planners in earlier periods (OECD 2003). This development is changing how many nations approach the relationship between government and society. Could not the United States join the vanguard of this international movement in the way it implements health reform?

This is not a rhetorical question given the harsh play of organizational and political forces within U.S. health policy. Analysts who monitor the public pulse on reform have observed: "The way in which the implementation process unfolds will affect the climate of public opinion at each stage, just as public opinion will, perhaps to a lesser degree, influence implementation going forward" (Brodie et al. 2010). Stated more forcefully: Public opinion will be a leading factor in the sustainability of health reform. Time is ripe for federal and state officials to align themselves with this reality.

Conclusion

Assessing the prospects for national health care reform from the vantage point of early 2009, Lawrence D. Brown imagined a spectrum of potential outcomes ranging from "fair and affordable universal coverage," at one extreme, to "a cruel charade" of insurance that is affordable or adequate but not both, at the other (Brown 2009: 4). "The devil, not yet in the details," he wrote, "haunts the design."

We are well beyond that point now. The die of national policy reform has been cast. Assuming President Obama's legislative success can survive the current political onslaught, the question becomes how will the countless *details of policy implementation* be handled? As with politics and policy formulation, the operational challenges of U.S. health care echo those found elsewhere around the world. Compiling a record of other nations' struggles may not offer great consolation for American observers, yet it just could help us approach our own administrative, regulatory, and planning responsibilities more nimbly than otherwise.

DISCUSSION QUESTIONS

1. Which aspects of the design of the Affordable Care Act do you think will be most challenging to implement?

2. Do you believe adoption of health reform by the United States will result in greater standardization or variation in the health systems of individual states? In your view, does this law make it time to "refigure" American federalism?
3. Will it be more feasible for the United States to learn from other nations' administrative practices than it has been to borrow from the design of their programs and laws?

VII: From Awareness to Utilization in Health Policy Learning

W riting shortly before passage of the Affordable Care Act, Trudy Rubin (2010), columnist for the *Philadelphia Inquirer*, observed: "One of the most bewildering aspects of the current health-care debate is the failure to learn key lessons from health systems abroad." Her puzzlement is understandable. The United States is afflicted with problems other nations have either solved or ameliorated to a great extent. Those accomplishments have been treated as peripheral in our process of health reform. The paradox is simply stated, not so an explanation. How can a public policy perspective shed light on this situation confusing even to a seasoned international reporter?

For policy studies specialists, learning lessons from abroad belongs to the broader subject known as "**policy transfer.**" According to the British scholar Diane Stone (1999: 51), policy transfer "is a dynamic whereby knowledge about policies, administrative arrangements or institutions is used across time or space in the development of policies, administrative arrangements and institutions elsewhere." The evidence is that policy transfer may be on the rise in our global era, particularly in parts of the world with strong regional links for economic development and other transnational issues. But policy transfer also assumes the form of practices migrating between completely different policy domains. **Privatization** is one example of a policy theme that has infiltrated a welter of program areas over time, both within and across nations. Competition is another whose potent influence has already been discussed in regard to contemporary approaches in health policy design.

It is not always easy to recognize when policy transfer has taken place across nations, or the precise degree to which it has taken place (Bennett 1997). Driving the policy process are many political forces and currents of information that can produce unexpected coincidence. Much easier is it to recognize when decision makers and advocates explicitly reject a particular foreign example, which is what has sometimes happened in U.S. health policy discourse. In his national address of September 2009, President Obama took pains to point out: "There are those on the left who believe that the only way to fix the system is through a single-payer system like Canada's, where we would severely restrict the private insurance market and have the government provide coverage for everyone." He then went on to discard this approach, characterizing it as a "radical shift" no more acceptable than the right-wing position of leaving "individuals to buy health insurance on their own."

As noted elsewhere in this book, international convergence in health care systems is evident. This phenomenon is progressing despite important national differences in public institutions and political culture. A main reason is the presence of overarching societal and industry factors inside the health sector, particularly in developed democracies, which show no respect for country boundaries. Among the most important pressures for convergence are population aging, the growing prevalence of chronic illnesses, rapid advances in medical technology, and rising public expectations and demands for treatment (Mechanic and Rochefort 1996). All these trends contribute to a need for increased health care access, cost-control, and quality improvement. Tackling these challenges, there are only so many policy tools of demonstrated effectiveness for nations to apply (Blank and Burau 2010).

Those who study policy transfer underscore the distinction between changes that are coercive versus voluntary in character. This is not so much about whether circumstances compel change within a country, but whether there is "imposition of a program, policy or institutional arrangement" from the outside (Dolowitz and Marsh 2000: 13). Coercion takes place when powerful nations or international organizations require states to conform to specified standards, provisions, and legal prescriptions as a condition for economic assistance or military protection. More indirectly, there are nations so hegemonic in the international community that their policy examples carry contagious weight due to the countries' status as role models coupled with exceptional ability to disseminate a preferred set of ideas (Dobbin, Simmons, and Garrett 2007). The United States is much more likely to be an *agent* than an *object* of coercion of this type. This customary position of dominance perhaps itself inhibits openness to the ideas and practices of other countries.

Voluntary policy transfer concerns situations in which national actors actively seek out information from other countries to address problems identified through a society's own political mechanisms. In other words, adoption of a foreign solution is willing, self-aware, and undertaken to satisfy the felt need for reform. Policy learning is the primary vehicle for voluntary policy transfer. There are several arguments, or hypotheses, about why it represents an integral part of an effective policy process (Stone 1999). First, rational policy making depends on a comprehensive search for information, and the collection of policy data from abroad is nothing if not a corrective against parochial investigation. Second, a "proclivity towards policy learning and lesson-drawing could assist decision-makers to respond more quickly or appropriately to crises" (Stone 1999: 53). Third, cross-national policy learning can allow officials confronting problems of an unprecedented nature to consider what has happened in other societies already familiar with the issue. Conceivably, it can even provide a basis for proactive decision-making fueled by well-reasoned assessment that a situation is "heading our way," as with an emerging pandemic or the advent of expensive new medical technologies and medicines.

Certainly, there is no shortage of information for an American audience about medicine and health policy in other countries. One need only peruse the content of major journals in this field—*Health Affairs, The Milbank Quarterly, Journal of Health Politics, Policy and Law, New England Journal of Medicine*, and others—to know this is true. During their coverage of the national health reform debate, the *New York Times* and *Washington Post* each published series on international health care developments. Similarly, leading foundations with an interest in health care such as The Kaiser Family Foundation, The Commonwealth Fund, and The Robert Wood Johnson Foundation all devote extensive space on their websites to international material. Even agencies of the United States government, such as the U.S. General Accounting Office (1991), have carried out cross-national analyses of health care. The crux of the issue of health policy learning, then, is not whether relevant evidence from other countries is available, nor whether there is awareness of this information among specialists, public officials, and well-informed members of the public. The question is what interferes with translation of this awareness into utilization within the policy process (Bennett 1991).

The mistake is regarding information about foreign programs as a set of neutral facts collected for dispassionate analysis within a framework of rational decision-making. More realistic is to recognize the highly politicized nature of the circumstances, and the fact that "political adversaries ... are using such lessons as political weapons" (Robertson 1991: 55). On one side, reform advocates solicit attention for selected foreign examples in raising the public profile of a problem and arguing the feasibility of a pre-conceived policy direction. On the other side, opponents may seize on this same example to generate "negative lessons to emphasize the risks of other polities' initiatives, to associate these programs with negative consequences and to highlight the unique features of their political system that make emulation unlikely to succeed" (Robertson 1991: 56).

Inevitably, this back-and-forth results in distortion, a shift from fact-based discussion to debate over values, and subsuming of the entire lesson-drawing exercise to habitual categories of ideological dispute. As positions on both sides harden and grow more extreme, an all-or-nothing discourse is prone to develop about particular national examples. This obscures the possibilities of picking and choosing more creatively across many nations, taking advantage of whatever elements of program design might be implemented as pragmatic responses to challenges here at home.

Powerful actors on the U.S. political scene stand ready to commit enormous resources to inflame such disagreements over foreign lesson drawing. When the filmmaker Michael Moore produces a freewheeling documentary like *Sicko* for the purpose of lampooning the shortcomings of U.S. health care while promoting Canada's single-payer system as an unblemished alternative, it is part of the problem, although the propagandistic aims are obvious enough. More insidious is the guerilla campaign waged by insurers unnerved by this message and intent on wholesale discrediting of the Canadian system in American eyes. Wendell Potter is a former public relations executive for CIGNA insurance company now turned whistle-blower on the industry and its hidden strategies of profit-maximization and political manipulation. As lawmakers in Vermont recently took steps toward adopting a version of single-payer health care, Potter called on his own experiences as insurance insider in predicting how insurers would likely respond (Huff 2011). Among the communication strategies he forecasted were:

- Development of an ad campaign against "government takeover" of health care
- Distribution of anti-single-payer messages and talking points to talk show producers and friendly members of Congress and the media
- Internet dissemination of vignettes of "victims" of single-payer health care
- Formation of alliances with conservative political groups also committed to quelling support for a Canadian-style system in the U.S.
- Efforts to build the impression of a grassroots backlash against the Vermont legislative proposal
- Commitment of resources for a broader political initiative to replace Vermont's governor and unfriendly members of the legislature in the next election cycle

Emphasizing the insurance industry's skills at deception in staging activities such as these, Potter stated: "You will not even be aware they're behind it."

It is a formidable wall of resistance to lesson learning that rises up when the mobilization of threatened interests combines with cultural skepticism about the relevance of what goes on elsewhere in the world. To return to an opening theme of this book, resistance of this kind is part and parcel of an "exceptionalist" belief system that sets the U.S. apart within the international community by valuing American institutions, social arrangements, and public philosophy as inherently different from, and above, all others (Kohut and Stokes 2006). Suspicion of foreign ideas is not just a static cultural disposition, however. Strength of reaction also seems proportional to the nature of the policy lessons under consideration. Political scientist James Morone (1990: 141) has attributed the limited impact of foreign lessons in U.S. health policy making to the fact that none of the big insights would be easy to adopt and implement given culturally accepted uses of public power in our society: "Instead of hard conscious choices, we have sought painless automatic solutions. Rather than explicit programmatic decisions Americans prefer hidden, implicit policies. Rather than centralize control in governmental hands, we would scatter it across many players."

Amid all constraints discussed here, are there any promising recommendations for learning from abroad in U.S. health policy making? A few ideas do merit mention as this book comes to a close.

First, we can focus more clearly on what we need to learn, scanning the international scene systematically with these objectives in mind. Even among policy analysts, policy advisors, and journalists, there are fads and fashions, as well as cultural biases, in the country examples deemed most significant. But the search for the "best" system is surely quixotic and, ultimately, distracting given varying expectations for health care from one society to another (Blank and Burau 2010). The object of learning should not be an entire system of care, so much as policy and program elements that can be abstracted from environment A and usefully adapted in environment B (Glaser 1993). We have talked about access, cost containment, and quality as dimensions of health system performance. Each can be broken down further according to operational areas within primary care, acute care, long-term care, public health, mental health services, and other major sectors of the health system. Sometimes the United States has drawn criticism for seeking technical fixes in health policy while avoiding difficult value choices. So long as those value choices remain controversial to the point of producing near paralysis, however, it seems reasonable to mold the lesson-drawing process around technical questions pursued and applied with narrow purposefulness.

Second, this instrumental approach to health policy learning means heightened "sensitivity towards the specific contexts under which policies succeed" (Blank and Burau 2010: 249). British health economist Barbara McPake (2002) has written about the difficulties of lesson-drawing on the African continent with respect to two health policy changes broadly applied or recommended cross-nationally, the introduction of user charges for health services and the movement for greater autonomy of public hospitals. In both cases, outcomes proved very disappointing: "The introduction of policies that may be seen to work well elsewhere, but which have been inadequately contextualized imposes serious costs, and in many cases may be worse than 'no change'" (p. 138). Discrepancies of context between developed and developing countries may be particularly pronounced in health reform, but they usefully dramatize an issue that, to a greater or lesser extent, arises in all cases of attempted policy learning. The designation of "best practices" will always be relative, not absolute, simply because it must factor in conditions inside both "exporting" and "importing" nations that bear on policy transfer through adaptation.

Third, more or less opportune time frames exist for attempting to learn policy lessons. Rudolf Klein (2009) offers astute advice on this matter. Be cautious of new developments, giving serious consideration only to policies having a long track record of demonstrated effectiveness in their home country. Look for policies already successful among several countries. Observe how other countries deal with the *process* of policy change, in particular the messy challenge of applying uncertain solutions within idiosyncratic political and organizational circumstances.

Policy learning should be seen as just another tool of government. It is not an end in itself, but rather a disposition and a procedure for enhancing the way health policy decisions get made. The only test that matters is whether policy learning works, that is, whether advantageous ideas from other countries can be identified, understood, adopted, and implemented in a way that generates concrete benefits. It is a rule most comparativists would be content to live by.

DISCUSSION QUESTIONS

1. How confident are you that health policy discourse in the United States can be altered to increase openness to lessons from abroad?
2. With the passage of time, do you think health care policies will continue to "converge" among different nations? Will the United States be a part of this trend?
3. Are you more concerned about the potential benefits or the pitfalls that might come with importing health policy ideas from other countries? How can policymakers maximize the former while minimizing the latter?
4. Ten years from now, what will be the state of health care in the United States?

References

Aaron, Henry J. 2010. "The Health Care Reform Battle Is Far from Over." Brookings Up Front Blog, October 8. Retrieved August 1, 2011 (http://www.brookings.edu/opinions/2010/1008_health_care_courts_aaron.aspx?comments=1).

Aaron, Henry J. 2011. "The Independent Payment Advisory Board—Congress's 'Good Deed.'" *New England Journal of Medicine* 364(25): 2377–79.

ABC News. 2010. "Transcript: GOP Response to State of the Union Address." January 27. Retrieved February 15, 2011 (http://abcnews.go.com/Politics/State_of_the_Union/state-of-the-union-bob-mcdonnell-gop-response-transcript/story?id=9673482).

Adolino, Jessica R. and Charles H. Blake. 2011. *Comparing Public Policies: Issues and Choices in Industrialized Countries*, 2nd edition. Washington, D.C.: CQ Press.

Agger, Ben. 2010. *Body Problems: Running and Living Long in a Fast-Food Society*. New York: Routledge.

Alford, Robert R. 1972. "The Political Economy of Health Care: Dynamics Without Change." *Politics & Society* 2: 127–64.

Anderson, James E. 2003. *Public Policymaking*, 5th edition. Boston: Houghton Mifflin.

Anderson, Odin W. 1963. "Medical Care: Its Social and Organizational Aspects: Health Services Systems in the United States and Other Countries." *New England Journal of Medicine* 269: 839–43.

Antonuccio, David O., David D. Burns, and William G. Danton. 2002. "Antidepressants: A Triumph of Marketing Over Science?" *Prevention & Treatment* 5: Article 25.

Appleby, Julie and Christopher Weaver. 2011. "After Much Scrutiny, HHS Releases Health Insurance Exchange Rules." Kaiser Health News, July 11. Retrieved August 1, 2011 (http://www.kaiserhealthnews.org/Stories/2011/July/11/Health-Insurance-Exchange-Regulations-Released.aspx).

Baker, Sam. 2011. "States Slow in Setting Up Central Piece of Obama Healthcare Law." Healthwatch, July 6. Retrieved August 1, 2011 (http://thehill.com/blogs/healthwatch/health-reform-implementation/169761-states-lag-in-implementing-health-insurance-exchanges).

Banting, Keith G. and Stan Corbett. 2002. "Health Policy and Federalism: An Introduction." Pp. 1–38 in *Health Policy and Federalism: A Comparative Perspective on Multi-Level Governance*, eds. Keith G. Banting and Stan Corbett. Montreal and Kingston: McGill-Queen's University Press.

Bardach, Eugene. 2009. *A Practical Guide for Policy Analysis: The Eightfold Path to More Effective Problem Solving*. Washington, D.C.: CQ Press.

Baumgartner, Frank R. and Bryan D. Jones. 1993. *Agendas and Instability in American Politics*. Chicago: University of Chicago Press.

Becker, Bernie and Jeff Zeleny. 2010. "Bayh Decides Against Re-election Bid." *New York Times*, February 15. Retrieved June 30, 2011 (http://thecaucus.blogs.nytimes.com/2010/02/15/bayh-decides-against-re-election-bid/).

Benelli, Eva. 2003. "The Role of the Media in Steering Public Opinion on Healthcare Issues." *Health Policy* 63(2): 179–86.

Bennett, Colin J. 1991. "How States Utilize Foreign Evidence." *Journal of Public Policy* 11(1): 31–54.

Bennett, Colin J. 1997. "Review Article: What Is Policy Convergence and What Causes It?" *British Journal of Political Science* 21(2): 215–33.

Bialik, Carl. 2009. "Ill-Conceived Ranking Makes for Unhealthy Debate." *Wall Street Journal*, October 21, p. A19.

Blank, Robert H. and Viola Burau. 2010. *Comparative Health Policy*, 3rd edition. New York: Palgrave Macmillan.

Bodenheimer, Thomas. 2003. "The American Health Care System: The Movement for Improved Quality in Health Care." Pp. 445–54 in *The Nation's Health*, 7th edition, eds. Philip R. Lee and Carroll L. Estes. Sudbury, MA: Jones and Bartlett Publishers.

Bodenheimer, Thomas. 2005. "High and Rising Health Care Costs. Part 3: The Role of Health Care Providers." *Annals of Internal Medicine* 142(12): 996–1002.

Brandon, William P., Rosemary V. Chaudry, and Alice Sardell. 2001. "Launching SCHIP: The States and Children's Health Insurance." Pp. 142–85 in *The New Politics of State Health Policy*, eds. Robert B. Hackey and David A. Rochefort. Lawrence: University Press of Kansas.

Brereton, Laura and Vilashiny Vasoodaven. 2010. "The Impact of the NHS Market: An Overview of the Literature." London: CIVITAS Institute for the Study of Civil Society.

Brodie, Mollyann, Drew Altman, Claudia Deane, Sasha Buscho, and Elizabeth Hamel. 2010. "Liking the Pieces, Not the Package: Contradictions in Public Opinion During Health Reform." *Health Affairs* 29(6): 1125–30.

Brown, Lawrence D. 2005. "Incrementalism Adds Up?" Pp. 315–35 in *Healthy, Wealthy, & Fair: Health Care and the Good Society*, eds. James A. Morone and Lawrence R. Jacobs. New York: Oxford University Press.

Brown, Lawrence D. 2009. *Refiguring Federalism: Nation and State in Health Reform's Next Round*. Washington, D.C.: National Academy of Social Insurance, January.

Brownson, Ross C., Tegan K. Boehmer, and Douglas A. Luke. 2005. "Declining Rates of Physical Activity in the United States: What Are the Contributors?" *Annual Review of Public Health* 26: 421–43.

Budrys, Grace. 2010. *Unequal Health: How Inequality Contributes to Health or Illness*, 2nd edition. Lanham, MD: Rowman & Littlefield Publishers.

Burau, Viola and Robert H. Blank. 2006. "Comparing Health Policy: An Assessment of Typologies of Health Systems." *Journal of Comparative Policy Analysis* 8(1): 63–76.

Busch, Susan H. and Colleen L. Barry. 2009. "Pediatric Antidepressant Use After the Black-Box Warning." *Health Affairs* 28(3): 724–33.

Callahan, Daniel. 2009. "Cost Control—Time to Get Serious." *New England Journal of Medicine* 361: e10. Retrieved April 30, 2011 (http://www.nejm.org/doi/full/10.1056/NEJMp0905630).

Carrin, Guy and Chris James. 2005. "Social Health Insurance: Key Factors Affecting the Transition towards Universal Coverage." *International Social Security Review* 58(1): 45–64. Retrieved April 30, 2011 (http://www.who.int/health_financing/documents/shi_key_factors.pdf).

Cauchi, Richard. 2011. "State Legislation and Actions Challenging Certain Health Reforms, 2011." National Conference of State Legislatures, June 29.

Centers for Medicare & Medicaid Services (CMS). 2010a. "2010 Actuarial Report on the Financial Outlook for Medicaid." December 21. Retrieved March 20, 2011 (http://www.cms.gov/ActuarialStudies/03_MedicaidReport.asp#TopOfPage).

Centers for Medicare & Medicaid Services (CMS). 2010b. "2010 Annual Report of the Board of Trustees of the Federal Hospital Insurance and Federal Supplementary Medical Insurance Trust Funds." August 5. Retrieved March 20, 2011 (http://www.cms.gov/ReportsTrustFunds/).

Centers for Medicare & Medicaid Services (CMS). 2010c. "CHIP 2010 Annual Enrollment Report." Retrieved March 20, 2011 (http://www.cms.gov/NationalCHIPPolicy/CHIPER/list.asp).

Chaddock, Gail Russell. 2009. "Health Care Reform: Obama Cut Private Deals with Likely Foes." *Christian Science Monitor*, November 6. Retrieved June 27, 2011 (http://www.csmonitor.com/USA/Politics/2009/1106/healthcare-reform-obama-cut-private-deals-with-likely-foes).

Chan, Margaret. 2009. "Addressing the Global Economic Crisis While Fighting Inequalities." WHO Office to the EU, April 3. Retrieved June 15, 2011 (http://pr.euractiv.com/press-release/addressing-global-economic-crisis-while-fighting-inequalities-9075?page=1).

Chinitz, David. 1995. "Israel's Health Policy Breakthrough: The Politics of Reform and the Reform of Politics." *Journal of Health Politics, Policy and Law* 20(4): 910–32.

Choudhry, Sujit and Benjamin Perrin. 2007. "The Legal Architecture of Intergovernmental Transfers: A Comparative Examination." Pp. 259–92 in *Intergovernmental Fiscal Transfers: Principles and Practice*, eds. Robin Boadway and Anwar Shah. Washington, D.C.: World Bank.

Cohn, Jonathan. 2011. "Yes, Let's Talk About Rationing." *The New Republic*, June 9. Retrieved August 1, 2011 (http://www.tnr.com/blog/jonathan-cohn/89722/ration-health-medicare-ryan-obamacare-brooks).

Contandriopoulos, Damien and Henriette Bilodeau. 2009. "The Political Use of Poll Results about Public Support for a Privatized Healthcare System in Canada." *Health Policy* 90(1): 104–12.

Crimmins, Eileen M., Samuel H. Preston, and Barney Cohen, eds. 2011. *Explaining Divergent Levels of Longevity in High-Income Countries*. Washington, D.C.: National Research Council.

Dahl, Espen and Marit Lie. 2009. "Policies to Tackle Health Inequalities in Norway: From Laggard to Pioneer?" *International Journal of Health Services* 39(3): 509–23.

Dahlgren, Göran and Margaret Whitehead. 1991. *Policies and Strategies to Promote Social Equity in Health*. Stockholm: Institute for Futures Studies.

Dahlgren, Göran and Margaret Whitehead. 1993. "Tackling Inequalities in Health: What Can We Learn from What has been Tried?" Working paper prepared for the King's Fund International Seminar on Tackling Inequalities in Health, September 1993, Ditchley Park, Oxfordshire. London: King's Fund.

Dahlgren, Göran and Margaret Whitehead. 2007. *European Strategies for Tackling Social Inequities in Health: Levelling up Part 2*. Copenhagen: WHO Regional office for Europe. (http://www.euro.who.int/__data/assets/pdf_file/0018/103824/E89384.pdf).

Daschle, Tom. 2010. *Getting it Done: How Obama and Congress Finally Broke the Stalemate to Make Way for Health Care Reform.* New York: St. Martin's Press.

Davis, Karen, Cathy Schoen, and Kristof Stremikis. 2010. "Mirror, Mirror on the Wall: How the Performance of the U.S. Health System Compares Internationally, 2010 Update." Commonwealth Fund, June 23. Retrieved February 15, 2011 (http://www.commonwealthfund.org/Content/Publications/Fund-Reports/2010/Jun/Mirror-Mirror-Update.aspx?page=all).

De Cock, Johan. 2002. "Federalism and the Belgian Health-Care System." Pp. 39–68 in *Health Policy and Federalism: A Comparative Perspective on Multi-Level Governance*, eds. Keith G. Banting and Stan Corbett. Montreal and Kingston: McGill-Queen's University Press.

Deber, Raisa. 2009. "Canada." Pp. 15–40 in *Cost Containment and Efficiency in National Health Systems: A Global Comparison*, eds. John Rapoport, Philip Jacobs, and Egon Jonsson. Weinheim, Germany: Wiley-VCH.

Dobbin, Frank, Beth Simmons, and Geoffrey Garrett. 2007. "The Global Diffusion of Public Policies: Social Construction, Coercion, or Learning?" *Annual Review of Sociology* 33: 449–72.

Docteur, Elizabeth and Robert A. Berenson. 2009. "How Does the Quality of U.S. Health Care Compare Internationally?" Robert Wood Johnson Foundation and Urban Institute, August 2009. Retrieved February 15, 2011 (http://www.rwjf.org/qualityequality/product.jsp?id=47508).

Docteur, Elizabeth and Howard Oxley. 2003. *Health-Care Systems: Lessons from the Reform Experience.* Paris: OECD Health Working Papers.

Dolowitz, David P. and David Marsh. 2000. "Learning from Abroad: The Role of Policy Transfer in Contemporary Policy-Making." *Governance* 13(1): 5–24.

Donohue, Julie M., Marisa Cevasco, and Meredith B. Rosenthal. 2007. "A Decade of Direct-to-Consumer Advertising of Prescription Drugs." *New England Journal of Medicine* 357: 673–81.

Eckstein, Harry. 1988. "A Culturalist Theory of Political Change." *American Political Science Review* 82(3): 789–804.

Engelhard, Carolyn L., Arthur Garson, Jr., and Stan Dorn. 2009. *Reducing Obesity: Strategies from the Tobacco Wars.* Washington, D.C.: The Urban Institute.

Entman, Robert M. 2004. *Projections of Power: Framing News, Public Opinion, and U.S. Foreign Policy.* Chicago: University of Chicago Press.

Esfandiari, Shahrokh. 2010. "The Limited Role of Citizens in Shaping Healthcare Policies." *World Medical and Health Policy* 2(1): 43–51.

Evans, Robert G. 2008. "Devil Take the Hindmost? Private Health Insurance and the Rising Costs of American 'Exceptionalism.'" Pp. 445–74 in *Health Politics and Policy*, 4th edition, eds. James A. Morone, Theodor J. Litman, and Leonard S. Robins. Clifton Park, NY: Delmar.

Farber, Dan. 2010. "Obama: We Can't Back Off Healthcare Reform." CBS News Political Hotsheet, February 7. Retrieved June 15, 2011 (http://www.cbsnews.com/8301-503544_162-6183917-503544.html).

Field, Mark G. 1973. "The Concept of the 'Health System' at the Macrosociological Level." *Social Science & Medicine* 7(10): 763–85.

Finkelstein, Eric A., Justin G. Trogdon, Joel W. Cohen, and William Dietz. 2009. "Annual Medical Spending Attributable To Obesity: Payer-And Service-Specific Estimates." *Health Affairs* 28(5): w822–w831.

Flegal, Katherine M., Margaret D. Carroll, Cynthia L. Ogden, and Lester R. Curtin. 2010. "Prevalence and Trends in Obesity among U.S. Adults, 1999–2008." *Journal of the American Medical Association* 303(3): 235–41.

Fox News. 2009. "Transcript: Economic Roundtable on 'FNS.'" June 8. Retrieved February 15, 2011 (http://www.foxnews.com/story/0,2933,525363,00.html).

Freeman, Richard. 1998. "Competition in Context: The Politics of Health Care Reform in Europe." *International Journal for Quality in Health Care* 10(5): 395–401.

Freeman, Richard and Lorraine Frisina. 2010. "Health Care Systems and the Problem of Classification." *Journal of Comparative Policy Analysis* 12(1&2): 163–78.

Friel, Sharon and Michael G. Marmot. 2011. "Action on the Social Determinants of Health and Health Inequities Goes Global." *Annual Review of Public Health* 32: 225–36.

Gamble, Vanessa Northington and Deborah A. Stone. 2006. "U.S. Policy on Health Inequities: The Interplay of Politics and Research." *Journal of Health Politics, Policy and Law* 31(1): 93–126.

Gamson, William A. and Andre Modigliani. 1989. "Media Discourse and Public Opinion on Nuclear Power: A Constructionist Approach." *The American Journal of Sociology* 95(1): 1–37.

Gauthier-Villars, David. 2009. "France Fights Universal Health Care's High Cost." *Wall Street Journal*, August 7, p. A1.

Gerber, Alan S. and Eric M. Patashnik. 2010. "Problem Solving in a Polarized Age: Comparative Effectiveness Research and the Politicization of Evidence-Based Medicine." *The Forum* 8(1), Article 3. Retrieved June 29, 2011 (http://www.bepress.com/forum/vol8/iss1/art3/).

Glaser, William A. 1993. "Universal Health Insurance That Really Works: Foreign Lessons for the United States." *Journal of Health Politics, Policy and Law* 18(3): 695–722.

Glied, Sherry. 2009. "Single Payer as a Financing Mechanism." *Journal of Health Politics, Policy and Law* 34(4): 594–615.

Godt, Paul J. 1987. "Confrontation, Consent, and Corporatism: State Strategies and the Medical Profession in France, Great Britain, and West Germany." *Journal of Health Politics, Policy and Law* 12(3): 459–79.

Goldman, T. R. 2011. "Legal Challenges to Health Reform." *Health Affairs* Health Policy Brief, July 8. Retrieved August 1, 2011 (http://www.healthaffairs.org/healthpolicybriefs/brief.php?brief_id=49).

Gould, Steven Jay. 1985. "The Median Isn't the Message." *Discover Magazine* 6 (June): 40–42.

Grantmakers in Health. 2007. "Knowledge to Action: Social and Environmental Determinants of Health." Retrieved March 10, 2011 (http://www.gih.org/topics3985/topics_show.htm?doc_id=466659&attrib_id=8498).

Gray, Gwendolyn. 1996. "Reform and Reaction in Australian Health Policy." *Journal of Health Politics, Policy and Law* 21(3): 587–615.

Gray, Gwendolyn. 2004. *The Politics of Medicare: Who Gets What, When and How.* Sydney: University of South Wales Press.

Ham, Chris and Mats Brommels. 1994. "Health Care Reform in The Netherlands, Sweden, and the United Kingdom." *Health Affairs* 13(5): 106–19.

Hancock, Linda. 2002. "Australian Intergovernmental Relations and Health." Pp. 107–42 in *Health Policy and Federalism: A Comparative Perspective on Multi-Level Governance*, eds. Keith G. Banting and Stan Corbett. Montreal and Kingston: McGill-Queen's University Press.

Harris, Gardiner. 2011. "Talk Doesn't Pay, So Psychiatry Turns Instead to Drug Therapy." *New York Times*, March 6, p. A1.

Harvard School of Public Health. 2008. "Most Republicans Think the U.S. Health Care System is the Best in the World. Democrats Disagree." Press Release, March 20. Retrieved February 15, 2011 (http://www.hsph.harvard.edu/news/press-releases/2008-releases/republicans-democrats-disagree-us-health-care-system.html).

Hayes, Katherine and Sara Rosenbaum. 2010. "Legal Challenges to the Affordable Care Act." Health Reform GPS, December 14. Retrieved August 1, 2011 (http://healthreformgps.org/resources/health-reform-and-the-constitutional-challenges).

Health Canada. 2011. "Canada's Health Care System." Retrieved April 30, 2011 (http://www.hc-sc.gc.ca/hcs-sss/pubs/system-regime/2011-hcs-sss/index-eng.php).

Helman, Cecil G. 2007. *Culture, Health, and Illness*, 5th edition. London: Hodder Arnold.

Henke, Klaus-Dirk, Margaret A. Murray, and Claudia Ade. 1994. "Global Budgeting in Germany: Lessons for the United States." *Health Affairs* 13(4): 7–21.

Hensley, Scott. 2011. "Americans Are Even Fatter Than Canadians." National Public Radio, March 2. Retrieved March 29, 2011 (http://www.npr.org/blogs/health/2011/03/02/134205145/americans-are-even-fatter-than-canadians).

Hiltzik, Michael. 2009. "Healthcare Ideas Losing Out to Ideology." *Los Angeles Times*, September 7. Retrieved June 27, 2011 (http://articles.latimes.com/2009/sep/07/business/fi-hiltzik7).

Himmelstein, David U., Deborah Thorne, Elizabeth Warren, and Steffie Woolhandler. 2009. "Medical Bankruptcy in the United States, 2007: Results of a National Study." *The American Journal of Medicine* 122(8): 741–46.

Hisashige, Akinori. 2009. "Japan." Pp. 157–82 in *Cost Containment and Efficiency in National Health Systems: A Global Comparison*, eds. John Rapoport, Philip Jacobs, and Egon Jonsson. Weinheim, Germany: Wiley-VCH.

Hobbs, Suzanne Havala. 2008. "Getting from Fat to Fit: The Role of Policy in the Obesity Disaster." *Law & Governance* 9(1): 8–21.

Holtz-Eakin, Douglas and Michael J. Ramlet. 2010. "Health Care Reform is Likely to Widen Federal Budget Deficits, Not Reduce Them." *Health Affairs* 29(6): 1136–41.

Horwitz, Allan V. 2010. "How an Age of Anxiety Became an Age of Depression." *The Milbank Quarterly* 88(1): 112–38.

Huff, Mel. 2011. "Whistleblower Says Insurers Will Try to Undermine Single-Payer." VTDigger.org, February 26. Retrieved July 15, 2011 (http://vtdigger.org/2011/02/26/story-video-whistleblower-says-insurers-will-try-to-undermine-single-payer/).

Hulse, Carl and Jackie Calmes. 2011. "Obama Urged to Act Quickly on Budget Agreement." *New York Times*, June 2, p. A15.

Ikegami, Naoki. 1991. "Japanese Health Care: Low Cost Through Regulated Fees." *Health Affairs* 10(3): 87–109.

Immergut, Ellen M. 1992. *Health Politics: Interests and Institutions in Western Europe*. New York: Cambridge University Press.

Institute of Medicine. 2001. *Crossing the Quality Chasm: A New Health System for the 21st Century*. Washington, D.C.: National Academy of Sciences.

International Obesity Taskforce (IOTF). 2010. Press Release, August 24. Retrieved March 10, 2011 (http://www.iaso.org/site_media/uploads/IOTF_Letter_to_coalition_PressRelease.pdf).

Jackson, Jeffrey L. 1997. "The German Health System: Lessons for Reform in the United States." *Archives of Internal Medicine* 157(2): 155–60.

Jacobs, Lawrence R. 1993. *The Health of Nations: Public Opinion and the Making of American and British Health Policy.* Ithaca: Cornell University Press.

Jacobs, Lawrence R. and Theda Skocpol. 2010. *Health Care Reform and American Politics: What Everyone Needs to Know.* New York: Oxford University Press.

Jacobs, Rowena and Maria Goddard. 2000. *Social Health Insurance Systems in European Countries.* York, U.K.: Centre for Health Economics, University of York.

Jacobson, Louis. 2011. "Insurance Commissioners Prepare for Health Care Policy Conflicts." *Governing.* Retrieved September 21, 2011 (http://www.governing.com/blogs/politics/Insurance-Commissioners-Prepare-for-Health-Care-Policy-Conflicts.html#).

Jia, H. and El Lubetkin. 2010. "Trends in Quality-Adjusted Life Years Lost Contributed By Smoking and Obesity." *American Journal of Preventive Medicine* 38(2): 138–44.

Jones, Jeffrey M. 2010. "Ratings of U.S. Healthcare Quality, Coverage Best in 10 Years." Princeton, Gallup, Inc., November 19. Retrieved April 30, 2011 (http://www.gallup.com/poll/144848/ratings-healthcare-quality-coverage-best-years.aspx).

Jost, Timothy Stoltzfus. 2001. "Private or Public Approaches to Insuring the Uninsured: Lessons from International Experience with Private Insurance." *New York University Law Review* 76(2): 419–93.

Jost, Timothy Stoltzfus. 2010. "Health Insurance Exchanges and the Affordable Care Act: Key Policy Issues." The Commonwealth Fund, pub. no. 1426, July. Retrieved August 1, 2011 (http://www.commonwealthfund.org/Content/Publications/Fund-Reports/2010/Jul/Health-Insurance-Exchanges-and-the-Affordable-Care-Act.aspx#citation).

Kaiser Family Foundation. 2009. "Cost Sharing for Health Care: France, Germany, and Switzerland." Menlo Park, CA. Retrieved April 30, 2011 (http://www.kff.org/insurance/upload/7852.pdf).

Kaiser Family Foundation. 2011a. "Focus on Health Reform: Summary of New Health Reform Law." Menlo Park, CA. Retrieved April 20, 2011 (http://www.kff.org/healthreform/8061.cfm).

Kaiser Family Foundation. 2011b. "Health Care Spending in the United States and Selected OECD Countries: April 2011." Menlo Park, CA. Retrieved April 30, 2011 (http://www.kff.org/insurance/snapshot/OECD042111.cfm).

Kaiser Health Tracking Poll. 2009. "Public Opinion on Health Care Issues." Retrieved June 20, 2011 (http://www.kff.org/kaiserpolls/posr042309pkg.cfm).

Katz, Neil. 2010. "Sarah Palin: Americans Have 'God-Given Right' to be Fat?" CBS News Healthwatch, November 30. Retrieved March 10, 2011 (http://www.cbsnews.com/8301-504763_162-20024104-10391704.html).

Kelley, Ed. 2007. "Health, Spending and the Effort to Improve Quality in OECD Countries: A Review of the Data." *Journal of the Royal Society for the Promotion of Health* 127(2): 64–71.

Kingdon, John. 1995. *Agendas, Alternatives, and Public Policies.* Boston: Little, Brown.

Kirkpatrick, David D. 2009. "White House Affirms Deal on Drug Cost." *New York Times*, August 6, p. A1.

Klein, Ezra. 2009. "When It Comes to Healthcare, the U.S., Britain and Canada Are Hurting." *Los Angeles Times*, April 7. Retrieved August 1, 2011 (http://articles.latimes.com/2009/apr/07/opinion/oe-klein7).

Klein, Rudolf. 1995. "Big Bang Health Care Reform—Does it Work?: The Case of Britain's 1991 National Health Service Reforms." *The Milbank Quarterly* 73(3): 299–377.

Klein, Rudolf. 2009. "Learning from Others and Learning from Mistakes: Reflections on Health Policy Making." Pp. 305–18 in *Comparative Studies and the Politics of Modern Medical Care*, eds. Theodore R. Marmor, Richard Freeman, and Kieke G. H. Okma. New Haven: Yale University Press.

Kliff, Sarah. 2010. "The Polling Contradiction." *Newsweek*, February 19. Retrieved June 23, 2011 (http://www.newsweek.com/id/233890).

Kohut, Andrew and Bruce Stokes. 2006. "The Problem of American Exceptionalism." Washington, D.C.: Pew Research Center, May 9. Retrieved July 15, 2011 (http://pewresearch.org/pubs/23/the-problem-of-american-exceptionalism).

Kutch, Jessica. 2010. "Hell Freezes Over: Rush Limbaugh Loves Union Hospitals and Socialized Medicine." SEIU Blog, January 4. Retrieved February 15, 2011 (http://www.seiu.org/2010/01/hell-freezes-over-rush-limbaugh-loves-union-hospitals-and-socialized-medicine.php#).

Land, Gary. 1982. "American Images of British Compulsory Health Insurance." Pp. 55–76 in *Compulsory Health Insurance: The Continuing American Debate*, eds. Ronald L. Numbers. Westport, CT: Greenwood Press.

Lawder, David. 2010. "Boehner Vows to Repeal Obama Healthcare Reforms." Reuters, November 3. Retrieved February 15, 2011 (http://www.reuters.com/article/2010/11/03/us-usa-elections-republicans-health-idUSTRE6A25DB20101103).

Le Grand, Julian. 2007. *The Other Invisible Hand: Delivering Public Services through Choice and Competition*. Princeton: Princeton University Press.

Lee, Sang-Yi, Chang-Bae Chun, Yong-Gab Lee, and Nam Kyu Seo. 2008. "The National Health Insurance System as One Type of New Typology: The Case of South Korea and Taiwan." *Health Policy* 85(1): 105–13.

Light, Paul. 1995. *Still Artful Work: The Continuing Politics of Social Security Reform*. New York: McGraw-Hill.

Lipset, Seymour Martin. 1996. *American Exceptionalism: A Double-Edged Sword*. New York: Norton.

Liptak, Adam. 2011. "Supreme Court is Asked to Rule on Health Care." *New York Times*, September 28, p. A1.

Longest, Beaufort B. 2003. "The Process of Public Policymaking: A Conceptual Model." Pp. 129–34 in *The Nation's Health*, 7th edition, eds. Philip R. Lee and Carroll L. Estes. Sudbury, MA: Jones and Bartlett Publishers.

Lubove, Roy. 1968. *The Struggle for Social Security: 1900–1935*. Cambridge: Harvard University Press.

Lundgren, Bernt. 2009. "Experiences from the Swedish Determinants-Based Public Health Policy." *International Journal of Health Services* 39(3): 491–507.

MacGillis, Alec. 2010. "Democratic Leaders Working to Win Over Abortion Opponents for Health-Care Reform." *Washington Post*, March 5. Retrieved June 7, 2011 (http://www.washingtonpost.com/wp-dyn/content/article/2010/03/04/AR2010030405040.html).

MacLeod, G. K. 1994. "Health Care Financing Reform in New Zealand." *Health Affairs* 13(4): 210–15.

Marmor, Theodore R. 1994. "Lessons from the Frozen North." Pp. 487–94 in *The Politics of Health Care Reform: Lessons from the Past, Prospects for the Future*, eds. James A. Morone and Gary S. Belkin. Durham: Duke University Press.

Marmor, Theodore R. 2000. *The Politics of Medicare*, 2nd edition. Hawthorne, NY: Aldine De Gruyter.

Marmor, Theodore R., Richard Freeman, and Kieke Okma. 2008. "Learning about Health Care from Other Countries." Pp. 475–80 in *Health Politics and Policy*, 4th edition, eds. James A. Morone, Theodor J. Litman, and Leonard S. Robins. Clifton Park, NY: Delmar.

Marmor, Theodore R., Richard Freeman, and Kieke G. H. Okma, eds. 2009. *Comparative Studies and the Politics of Modern Medical Care*. New Haven: Yale University Press.

Marmor, Theodore R. and Jerry L. Mashaw. 1994. "Canada's Health Insurance and Ours: The Real Lessons, the Big Choices." Pp. 69–84 in *National Health Care*, ed. Jonathan Lemco. Ann Arbor: The University of Michigan Press.

Marmor, Theodore R. and Jonathan Oberlander. 1998. "Rethinking Medicare Reform." *Health Affairs* 17(1): 52–68.

Marmot, Michael. 2005. "Social Determinants of Health Inequalities." *Lancet* 365: 1099–104.

Mathews, Anna Wilde. 2011. "States Get Leeway on Shape of New Insurance Exchanges." *Wall Street Journal*, July 12. Retrieved August 1, 2011 (http://online.wsj.com/article/SB1000142405270230 458440457644032303486 7608.html).

McDonough, John E., Brian Rosman, Fawn Phelps, and Melissa Shannon. 2006. "The Third Wave of Massachusetts Health Care Access Reform." *Health Affairs* 25(6): w420–w431.

McPake, Barbara. 2002. "The Globalisation of Health Sector Reform Policies: Is 'Lesson Drawing' Part of the Process?" Pp. 120–39 in *Health Policy in a Globalising World*, eds. Kelley Lee, Kent Buse and Suzanne Fustukian. Cambridge: Cambridge University Press.

Mechanic, David. 1997. "Muddling Through Elegantly: Finding the Proper Balance in Rationing." *Health Affairs* 16(5): 83–92.

Mechanic, David and David A. Rochefort. 1996. "Comparative Medical Systems." *Annual Review of Sociology* 22: 239–70.

Mertens, Maggie. 2010. "Some Will Remain Uninsured After Reform." Kaiser Health News, March 24. Retrieved April 4, 2011 (http://www.kaiserhealthnews.org/Stories/2010/March/24/Some-Will-Remain-Uninsured.aspx).

Moran, Michael. 2000. "Understanding the Welfare State: The Case of Health Care." *British Journal of Politics & International Relations* 2(2): 135–60.

Morone, James A. 1990. "American Political Culture and the Search for Lessons from Abroad." *Journal of Health Politics, Policy and Law* 15(1): 129–43.

Morone, James A. 2008. "Introduction: Health Politics and Policy." Pp. 1–22 in *Health Politics and Policy*, 4th edition, eds. James A. Morone, Theodore J. Litman, and Leonard S. Robins. Clifton Park, NY: Delmar.

Mossialos, Elias and Julian Le Grand. 1999. "Cost Containment in the EU: An Overview." Pp. 1–154 in *Health Care and Cost Containment in the European Union*, eds. Elias Mossialos and Julian Le Grand. Aldershot, England: Ashgate.

Nathanson, Constance. 2005. "Interest Groups and the Reproduction of Inequality." Pp. 177–204 in *Healthy, Wealthy & Fair: Health Care and the Good Society*, eds. James A. Morone and Lawrence R. Jacobs. New York: Oxford University Press.

National Institute for Health and Clinical Excellence (NICE). 2009. *Depression: The Treatment and Management of Depression in Adults*. NICE Clinical Guideline 90. London.

National Public Radio (NPR). 2011. "Party Politics and the American Disconnect." *On Point with Tom Ashbrook*, May 11. Retrieved June 16, 2011 (http://onpoint.wbur.org/2011/05/11/party-politics-disconnect).

New York Times. 2011. "The Republican Debate at the Reagan Library." A transcription of the 2012 Republican presidential debate on Sept. 7, 2011, in Simi Valley, Calif., as transcribed by Roll Call. Retrieved September 9, 2011 (http://www.nytimes.com/2011/09/08/us/politics/08republican-debate-text.html?pagewanted=all).

Nielsen. 2009. "Average TV Viewing for 2008–09 TV Season." November 10. Retrieved March 10, 2011 (http://blog.nielsen.com/nielsenwire/media_entertainment/average-tv-viewing-for-2008-09-tv-season-at-all-time-high/).

Obama, Barack. 2009. "Remarks by the President to a Joint Session of Congress on Health Care." Washington, D.C., September 9. Retrieved March 21, 2011 (http://www.whitehouse.gov/the_press_office/remarks-by-the-president-to-a-joint-session-of-congress-on-health-care/).

Obama, Barack. 2010. "Remarks by the President and Vice President on Health Insurance Reform at the Department of the Interior." Washington, D.C., March 23. Retrieved March 21, 2011 (http://www.whitehouse.gov/the-press-office/remarks-president-and-vice-president-health-insurance-reform-bill-department-interi).

OBAMACARE Repeal Pledge. 2011. "The Repeal Pledge (Candidate's Version)." Retrieved August 1, 2011 (http://www.therepealpledge.com/the-repeal-pledge-candidate-version).

Okma, Kieke G. H., Tsung-Mei Cheng, David Chinitz, Luca Crivelli, Meng-Kin Lim, Hans Maarse, and Maria Eliana Labra. 2010. "Six Countries, Six Health Reform Models? Health Care Reform in Chile, Israel, Singapore, Switzerland, Taiwan, and The Netherlands." *Journal of Comparative Policy Analysis* 12(1–2): 75–113.

Okma, Kieke G. H. and Aad A. de Roo. 2009. "The Netherlands: From Polder Model to Modern Management." Pp. 120–52 in *Comparative Studies & the Politics of Modern Medical Care*, eds. Theodore R. Marmor, Richard Freeman, and Kieke G. H. Okma. New Haven: Yale University Press.

Organisation for Economic Co-operation and Development (OECD). 1987. *Financing and Delivering Health Care: A Comparative Analysis of OECD Countries*. Paris.

Organisation for Economic Co-operation and Development (OECD). 2001a. *Citizens as Partners: OECD Handbook on Information, Consultation and Public Participation in Policy-Making*. Paris.

Organisation for Economic Co-operation and Development (OECD). 2001b. "Engaging Citizens in Policy-Making: Information, Consultation and Public Participation." *OECD Public Management Brief*, July. Retrieved August 1, 2011 (http://www.oecd.org/dataoecd/24/34/2384040.pdf).

Organisation for Economic Co-operation and Development (OECD). 2003. "Engaging Citizens Online for Better Policy-Making." *Policy Brief*, March. Retrieved August 1, 2011 (http://www.oecd.org/dataoecd/62/23/2501856.pdf).

Organisation for Economic Co-operation and Development (OECD). 2004. "Proposal for a Taxonomy of Health Insurance." Pp. 1–21 in *OECD Health Project*. Paris.

Organisation for Economic Co-operation and Development (OECD). 2010. *Obesity and the Economics of Prevention: Fit Not Fat*. Paris.

Organisation for Economic Co-operation and Development (OECD). 2011. OECD Health Data, June 30, 2011. Retrieved September 23, 2011 (http://stats.oecd.org/Index.aspx?DataSetCode=SHA).

Orszag, Peter R. and Ezekiel J. Emanuel. 2010. "Health Care Reform and Cost Control." *New England Journal of Medicine* 363(7): 601–603. Retrieved June 10, 2011 (http://www.nejm.org/doi/pdf/10.1056/NEJMp1006571?ssource=hcrc).

Oxley, Howard and Maitland MacFarlan. 1995. "Health Care Reform: Controlling Spending and Increasing Efficiency." *OECD Economic Studies* 24.

Palin, Sarah. 2009. "Obama and the Bureaucratization of Health Care." *Wall Street Journal*, September 8. Retrieved August 1, 2011 (http://online.wsj.com/article/SB10001424052970203440104574400581157986024.html).

Patel, Kant and Mark Rushefsky. 2006. *Health Care Politics and Policy in America* 3rd edition. Armonk, NY: M.E. Sharpe.

Patient Protection and Affordable Care Act (H.R. 3590). 2010. Retrieved March 20, 2011 (http://democrats.senate.gov/pdfs/reform/patient-protection-affordable-care-act-as-passed.pdf).

Payer, Lynne. 1988. *Medicine and Culture: Varieties of Treatment in the United States, England, West Germany, and France*. New York: Penguin Books.

Payer, Lynne. 1990. "Borderline Cases: How Medical Practice Reflects National Culture." *Sciences* 30(4): 38–42.

Pear, Robert. 2002. "Investigators Find Repeated Deception in Ads for Drugs." *New York Times*, December 4. Retrieved March 10, 2011 (http://www.nytimes.com/2002/12/04/us/investigators-find-repeated-deception-in-ads-for-drugs.html).

Pear, Robert. 2010. "Health Insurance Companies Try to Shape Rules." *New York Times*, May 16, p. A22.

Pear, Robert. 2011. "Health Law to be Revised by Ending a Program." *New York Times*, October 14, p. A10.

Pearson, Mark. 2009. "Written Statement to Senate Special Committee on Aging." Paris: Organisation for Economic Co-operation and Development.

Peters, B. Guy. 2004. *American Public Policy: Promise and Performance*, 6th edition. Washington, D.C.: CQ Press.

Peterson, Mark. 2008. "Congress." Pp. 72–94 in *Health Politics and Policy*, 4th edition, eds. James A. Morone, Theodor J. Litman, and Leonard S. Robins. Clifton Park, NY: Delmar.

Public Law 93-641, Sec. 2(a)(1) 1975. "National Health Planning and Resources Development Act of 1974." Retrieved April 30, 2011 (http://www.cq.com/graphics/sal/93/sal93-641.pdf).

Puska, Pekka and Timo Ståhl. 2010. "Health in All Policies – The Finnish Initiative: Background, Principles, and Current Issues." *Annual Review of Public Health* 31: 315–28.

Pye, Lucien. 1968. "Political Culture." Pp. 218–24 in *International Encyclopedia of the Social Sciences*, eds. David L. Sills and Robert K. Merton. New York: Crowell Collier and Macmillan, Inc.

Quah, Stella. 2010. "Health and Culture." Pp. 27–46 in *The New Blackwell Companion to Medical Sociology*, ed. William C. Cockerham. Oxford, UK: Wiley-Blackwell.

Quincy, Lynn. 2011. "Making Health Insurance Cost-Sharing Clear to Consumers: Challenges in Implementing Health Reform's Insurance Disclosure Requirements." New York: The Commonwealth Fund.

Rapoport, John, Egon Jonsson, and Philip Jacobs. 2009. "Introduction and Summary." Pp. 1–14 in *Cost Containment and Efficiency in National Health Systems: A Global Comparison*, eds. John Rapoport, Philip Jacobs, and Egon Jonsson. Weinheim, Germany: Wiley-VCH.

Reagan, Michael D. 1999. *The Accidental System: Health Care Policy in America*. Boulder, CO: Westview Press.

Reid, T. R. 2009. *The Healing of America: A Global Quest for Better, Cheaper, and Fairer Health Care*. New York: The Penguin Press.

Reinhardt, Uwe E. 1980. "Health Insurance and Cost-Containment Policies: The Experience Abroad." *American Economic Review* 70(2): 149–56.

Reinhardt, Uwe E. 2009. "Health Reform without a Public Plan: The German Model." *New York Times*, April 17. Retrieved April 30, 2011 (http://economix.blogs.nytimes.com/2009/04/17/health-reform-without-a-public-plan-the-german-model/).

Robertson, David Brian. 1991. "Political Conflict and Lesson-Drawing." *Journal of Public Policy* 11(1): 55–78.

Robinson, James C. 2002. "Renewed Emphasis on Consumer Cost Sharing in Health Insurance Benefit Design." *Health Affairs Web Exclusive*, March 20. Retrieved May 24, 2011 (http://www.healthaffairs.org/RWJ/2103Robinson.pdf).

Rochefort, David A. 2001. "The Backlash against Managed Care." Pp. 113–41 in *The New Politics of State Health Policy*, eds. Robert B. Hackey and David A. Rochefort. Lawrence: University Press of Kansas.

Rochefort, David A. and Roger W. Cobb, eds. 1994. *The Politics of Problem Definition: Shaping the Policy Agenda*. Lawrence: University Press of Kansas.

Rochefort, David A. and Kevin P. Donnelly. 2008. "The Changing Influence of the Canadian Single-Payer Model in America's National Healthcare Debate." *Harvard Health Policy Review* 9(1): 132–48.

Rodwin, Victor G. 1987. "American Exceptionalism in the Health Sector: The Advantages of 'Backwardness' in Learning from Abroad." *Medical Care Review* 44(1): 119–54.

Rodwin, Victor G. 2003. "The Health Care System Under French National Health Insurance: Lessons for Health Reform in the United States." *American Journal of Public Health* 93(1): 31–7.

Roemer, Milton I. 1960. "Health Departments and Medical Care—A World Scanning." *American Journal of Public Health* 50(2): 154–60.

Rogne, Leah, Carroll Estes, Brian R. Grossman, and Brooke Hollister. 2009. *Social Insurance and Social Justice: Social Security, Medicare, and the Campaign Against Entitlements*. New York: Springer.

Ros, Corina C., Peter P. Groenewegen, and Diana M. J. Delnoij. 2000. "All Rights Reserved, or Can We Just Copy? Cost Sharing Arrangements and Characteristics of Health Care Systems." *Health Policy* 52(1): 1–13.

Rubin, Trudy. 2010. "U.S. Could Learn from Health Care Abroad." *Columbus Dispatch*, March 3. Retrieved July 15, 2011 (http://www.dispatch.com/live/content/editorials/stories/2010/03/03/u-s--could-learn-from-health-care-abroad.html).

Rutenberg, Jim and Jackie Calmes. 2009. "False 'Death Panel' Rumor Has Some Familiar Roots." *New York Times*, August 14, p. A1.

Saltman, Richard B., Reinhard Busse, and Josep Figueras, eds. 2004. *Social Health Insurance Systems in Western Europe*. Berkshire, England: Open University Press.

Saltman, Richard B. and Josep Figueras. 1998. "Analyzing the Evidence on European Health Care Reforms." *Health Affairs* 17(2): 85–108.

Schlesinger, Mark and Jacob S. Hacker. 2007. "Secret Weapon: 'The New' Medicare as a Route to Health Security." *Journal of Health Politics, Policy and Law* 32(2): 247–91.

Schlosser, Eric. 2005. *Fast Food Nation: The Dark Side of the All-American Meal*. New York: Harper Perennial.

Schneider, Anne and Helen Ingram. 1988. "Systematically Pinching Ideas: A Comparative Approach to Policy Design." *Journal of Public Policy* 8(1): 61–80.

Schoen, Cathy, Robin Osborn, Sabrina K. H. How, Michelle M. Doty, and Jordan Peugh. 2008. "In Chronic Condition: Experiences of Patients with Complex Health Care Needs, In Eight Countries, 2008." *Health Affairs Web Exclusive* 28(1): w1–w16.

Shields, Margot, Margaret D. Carroll, and Cynthia L. Ogden. 2011. "Adult Obesity Prevalence in Canada and the United States." *NCHS Data Brief*, no. 56, March. Retrieved March 10, 2011 (http://www.cdc.gov/nchs/data/databriefs/db56.pdf).

Sidel, Victor W. and Ruth Sidel. 1983. *A Healthy State: An International Perspective on the Crisis in United States Medical Care*, revised and updated ed. New York: Pantheon Books.

Skinner, Brett J. and Mark Rovere. 2010. "Value for Money from Health Insurance Systems in Canada and the OECD." Calgary, AB: Fraser Institute.

Sommers, Benjamin D. and Sara Rosenbaum. 2011. "Issues in Health Reform: How Changes in Eligibility May Move Millions Back and Forth between Medicaid and Insurance Exchanges." *Health Affairs* 30(2): 228–36.

Soroka, Stuart. 2007. "Canadian Perceptions of the Health Care System." Toronto: Health Council of Canada.

Staff of *The Washington Post*. 2010. *Landmark: The Inside Story of America's New Health-Care Law and What it Means for Us All*. New York: Public Affairs.

Stolberg, Sheryl Gay and Robert Pear. 2010. "Obama Signs Health Care Overhaul Bill, With a Flourish." *New York Times*, March 24, p. A19.

Stolberg, Sheryl Gay and Jeff Zeleny. 2009. "Obama, Armed with Details, Says Health Plan is Necessary." *New York Times*, September 10, p. A1.

Stone, Deborah A. 1981. "Drawing Lessons from Comparative Health Research." Pp. 135–48 in *Critical Issues in Health Policy*, eds. Ralph A. Straetz, Marvin Lieberman, and Alice Sardell. Lexington, MA: D.C. Heath.

Stone, Deborah A. 2001. *Policy Paradox: The Art of Political Decision Making*, 3rd edition. New York: Norton.

Stone, Diane. 1999. "Learning Lessons and Transferring Policy Across Time, Space and Disciplines." *Politics* 19(1): 51–9.

Stone, Peter H. 2010. "Health Insurers Funded Chamber Attack Ads." *National Journal*, January 12. Retrieved June 29, 2011 (http://undertheinfluence.nationaljournal.com/2010/01/health-insurers-funded-chamber.php).

Szabo, Liz. 2009. "Number of Americans Taking Antidepressants Doubles." *USA Today*, August 4. Retrieved March 29, 2011 (http://www.usatoday.com/news/health/2009-08-03-antidepressants_N.htm).

Tantaros, Andrea. 2011. "Obama's Death Panels Return: Rationing is at Heart of President's Health Plan." *New York Daily News*, May 12. Retrieved August 1, 2011 (http://articles.nydailynews.com/2011-05-12/news/29550087_1_cancer-patients-affordable-care-act-health-care).

Thomma, Steven. 2011. "Poll: Best Way to Fight Deficits: Raise Taxes on the Rich." *McClatchy Newspapers*, April 18. Retrieved June 1, 2011 (http://www.mcclatchydc.com/2011/04/18/112386/poll-best-way-to-fight-deficits.html).

Truman, Benedict I. et al. 2011. "Rationale for Regular Reporting on Health Disparities and Inequalities—United States." *Morbidity and Mortality Weekly Report* 60, Supplement, January 14.

Trust for America's Future and Robert Wood Johnson Foundation. 2010. *F as in Fat: How Obesity Threatens America's Future*. Washington, D.C.

Tuohy, Carolyn Hughes. 2009. "Canada: Health Care Reform in Comparative Perspective." Pp. 61–87 in *Comparative Studies and the Politics of Modern Medical Care*, eds. Theodore R. Marmor, Richard Freeman, and Kieke G. H. Okma. New Haven: Yale University Press.

Twaddle, Andrew C. 2002. *Health Care Reform Around the World*. Westport, CT: Greenwood Publishing.

U.S. Census Bureau. 2010. "Income, Poverty, and Health Insurance Coverage in the United States: 2009." Retrieved May 3, 2011 (http://www.census.gov/prod/2010pubs/p60-238.pdf).

U.S. Department of Health and Human Services. 2011. "National Strategy for Quality Improvement in Health Care." March. Washington, D.C. Retrieved April 30, 2011 (http://www.healthcare.gov/center/reports/nationalqualitystrategy032011.pdf).

U.S. General Accounting Office. 1991. *Canadian Health Insurance: Lessons for the United States*. HRD-91-90. Washington, D.C.

Visscher, Tommy L. S. and Jacob C. Seidell. 2001. "The Public Health Impact of Obesity." *Annual Review of Public Health* 22: 355–75.

Wasem, Jürgen and Stefan Greß. 2009. "Regulating Private Health Insurance Markets." Pp. 203–43 in *Comparative Studies and the Politics of Modern Medical Care*, eds. Theodore R. Marmor, Richard Freeman, and Kieke G. H. Okma. New Haven: Yale University Press.

Weil, Alan and Raymond Scheppach. 2010. "New Roles for States in Health Reform Implementation." *Health Affairs* 29(6): 1178–82.

Weil, Alan, Jacqueline Scott, Anne Gauthier, and Sonya Schwartz. 2009. "Supporting State Policymakers' Implementation of Health Reform." *State Health Policy Briefing*, National Academy for State Health Policy, November. Retrieved August 1, 2011 (http://www.nashp.org/node/1608).

Weisman, Jonathan. 2009. "Obama Used Faulty Anecdote in Speech to Congress." *Wall Street Journal*, September 17, p. A4.

Weissert, Carol S. and William G. Weissert. 2006. *Governing Health: The Politics of Health Policy*, 3rd edition. Baltimore: Johns Hopkins University Press.

Whitaker, Robert. 2010. *Mad in America: Bad Science, Bad Medicine, and the Enduring Mistreatment of the Mentally Ill*, 2nd edition. New York: Basic Books.

White, Joseph. 1995. *Competing Solutions: American Health Care Proposals and International Experience*. Washington, D.C.: The Brookings Institution.

Whitehead, Margaret and Göran Dahlgren. 2007. *Concepts and Principles for Tackling Social Inequities in Health: Leveling Up Part 1.* Copenhagen, Denmark: World Health Organization Regional Office for Europe.

White House. 2010. "The Affordable Care Act—Implementation Timeline." Retrieved May 5, 2011 (http://www.whitehouse.gov/healthreform/timeline).

Whitman, Glen. 2008. "Who's Fooling Who: The World Health Organization's Problematic Ranking of Health Care Systems." Briefing Paper no. 101, Cato Institute, February 28.

WHO World Mental Health Consortium. 2004. "Prevalence, Severity, and Unmet Need for Treatment of Mental Disorders in the World Health Organization World Mental Health Survey." *Journal of the American Medical Association* 291(21): 2581–90.

Wilkinson, Richard and Kate Picket. 2010. *The Spirit Level: Why Greater Equality Makes Societies Stronger.* New York: Bloomsbury Press.

Wilsford, David. 1991. *Doctors and the State: The Politics of Health Care in France and The United States.* Durham: Duke University Press.

World Health Organization (WHO). 2000. "World Health Organization Assesses the World's Health Systems." Retrieved February 15, 2011 (http://www.who.int/whr/2000/media_centre/press_release/en/).

World Health Organization (WHO). 2008. *Closing the Gap in a Generation: Health Equity through Action on the Social Determinants of Health.* Final Report of the Commission on the Social Determinants of Health. Geneva: WHO Press.

World Health Organization (WHO). 2010a. *Adelaide Statement on Health in All Policies: Moving Towards a Shared Governance for Health and Well-Being.* Report from the International Meeting on Health in All Policies, Adelaide. Geneva: WHO Press.

World Health Organization (WHO). 2010b. *World Health Statistics 2010.* Geneva: WHO Press.

World Health Organization (WHO) and World Organization of Family Doctors (Wonca). 2008. *Integrating Mental Health into Primary Care: A Global Perspective.* Geneva: WHO Press.

Wörz, Markus and Reinhard Busse. 2009. "Germany." Pp. 97–130 in *Cost Containment and Efficiency in National Health Systems: A Global Comparison*, eds. John Rapoport, Philip Jacobs, and Egon Jonsson. Weinheim, Germany: Wiley-VCH.

Zaharoff, Josh. 2009. "Legislating Under the Influence." Common Cause, June 24. Retrieved July 1, 2011 (http://www.commoncause.org/atf/cf/%7Bfb3c17e2-cdd1-4df6-92be-bd4429893665%7D/COMMON_CAUSE_HEALTHCAREREPORT_JUNE2009.PDF).

Glossary/Index

Belgium 49, 61–2

Benelli, Eva 43

Bennett, Colin 69, 71

Berenson, Robert 2

best practices: methods or techniques generally regarded as being most effective in achieving a desired outcome 56, 73

Bialik, Carl 3

big bang policy: legislation that involves system-wide change and a dramatic departure from the status quo 37-38

Bilodeau, Henriette 43

Blair, Tony 9, 53

Blake, Charles 60

Blank, Charles 4, 8, 10, 51, 64, 65, 70, 73

Blank, Robert 22

Bodenheimer, Thomas 51, 55

Boehmer, Tegan 25

Boehner, John 1, 58

Brandeis, Justice 15

Brandon, William 15

Brazil 26

Brereton, Laura 53

Brodie, Mollyann 67

Brommels, Mats 64

Brown, Lawrence 39, 63, 67

Brownson, Ross 25

budgetary restraints on health care policy 43–4

Budrys, Grace 28

Burau, Viola 4, 8, 10, 22, 51, 64, 65, 70, 73

Burns, David 24

Busch, Susan 24

Busse, Reinhard 49, 52

C

Cain, Herman xi

Callahan, Daniel 55

Calmes, Jackie 44, 63

Canada 4, 54

    buying power 51

    health policy 48, 61, 64

    public opinion 43

Canadian Centre for Social Justice 29

Carrin, Guy 48, 49

Carroll, Estes 25

Cauchi, Richard 59

Centers for Disease Control 25, 30–1

Cevasco, Marisa 23

Chaddock, Gail 36

Chan, Margaret 44

Chaudry, Rosemary 15

checks and balances: a principle of the American political system whereby each branch of government is empowered to amend or block the actions of the others 35

Chile 66

Chinitz, David 41

CHIP *see* **State Children's Health Insurance Program**

Choudhry, Sanjit 62

classification of national health systems 7–10

Clinton, Bill 34, 52

CMS 14, 15

Cobb, Roger 10

Cohen, Barney 3

Cohn, Jonathan 63

Commission to Build a Healthier America 30

Commonwealth Fund 2–3, 63, 71

community health centers 13, 17

competition: a health policy strategy that requires providers or insurers to strive for better performance in fulfilling specified health care goals while rewarding that performance with financial incentives or the promise of greater market share 9–10, 52–4

Contandriopoulos, Damien 43

convergence: a theory that suggests health care policies and services are becoming increasingly similar across nations because of growing commonality of health system pressures such as illness patterns, rising costs, technology advances, and other factors 56, 70

copayment: a flat fee paid out-of-pocket per episode of medical service 14, 54

Corbett, Stan 61, 62

cost sharing: an insurance or health policy provision that requires subscribers to pay a portion of service costs, such as a deductible or copayment 54–5

costs 11–13

    containment in private insurance 13–14

    fostering monopsony to control 51–2

    and funding of ACA 17–18, 55

Entman, Robert 34

epidemic: a disease or medical condition that is extremely widespread, affecting many people at the same time 24

Esfandiari, Shahrokh 66

Evans, Robert 51

evidence-based medicine: the practice of using the best available evidence from clinical outcomes to inform decisions regarding the treatment of individual patients 40, 64

exceptionalism 3, 72

F

F as in Fat 26

Farber, Dan 45

federal systems *see* **federalism**

federalism: a system of government in which authority is divided between a centralized governing body and regional or state governments 60–3

Field, Mark 7–8

Figueras, Josep 49, 54

filibustering: a legislative maneuver within the U.S. Senate in which the minority party blocks a measure from coming up for floor vote by refusing to close debate; the majority party can only overcome a filibuster when it controls three-fifths of votes in the body 37

Finkelstein, Eric 25

Finland 30

Flegal, Katherine 25

France
    cost sharing 54
    health expenditure 51
    incremental health reform in 38
    medicine in 21
    reductions in health services 44

Freeman, Richard 3, 4, 10, 54

Friel, Sharon 30

Frisina, Lorraine 10

G

Galston, William 39

Gamble, Vanessa 31

Gamson, William 34

Garrett, Geoffrey 70

Garson, Arthur 26

Gauthier-Villars, David 44
GDP, health spending as a percentage of 12, 50–1
Gerber, Alan 40
Germany 4, 21, 22, 54
    health care policy 9, 49, 53
    single-payer system 51–2
Glaser, William 48, 73
Glied, Sherry 52
Goddard, Maria 49, 53
Godt, Paul 34
Goldman, T.R. 59, 60
Gould, Stephen Jay 27
Gray, Gwendolyn 39, 40
Greece 9
Greß, Stefan 66
Groenewegen, Peter 54

H
Hacker, Jacob 15
Ham, Chris 64
Hancock, Linda 61
Harris, Gardiner 23
Harvard School of Public Health 2
Hayes, Katherine 60
Health Affairs 60
Health Care Quality Indicators project 56
health care quality: the degree to which health services are clinically appropriate,
    delivered and utilized in an appropriate manner, and achieve desired health out-
    comes 2–3, 55–6
health care reform: an attempt to improve health system performance through pub-
    lic policy, typically centered around issues of access, cost, and quality 4
    battles over ACA 35–7
    and budgetary shortfall 43–4
    ideology versus problem solving 39–40
    incremental and innovative legislative reforms 37–9
    policy process 33–5
    and public opinion 42–3
    and public participation 66–7
    and special interest groups 34, 36, 40–2, 65
health disparities: differences in health indicators across subgroups of a population
    2, 26–8

health inequities: differences in health indicators across subgroups of a population that are considered to be avoidable and/or unfair 28–31

health insurance exchange: a government or quasi-government entity that offers health insurance consumers a range of coverage options from competing health insurers; State-run exchanges are a central part of the 2010 U.S. Affordable Care Act 16–17, 54, 62, 65

health measures, comparative 26, 27

health spending as a percentage of GDP 12, 50–1

A Healthy State 4

Helman, Cecil 20

Henke, Klaus-Dirk 49

Hensley, Scott 25

Hiltzik, Michael 39

Himmelstein, David 12

Hisashige, Akinori 52

Hobbs, Suzanne Havala 25

Holtz-Eakin, Douglas 18

Horwitz, Allan 23

Huff, Mel 72

Hulse, Carl 44

I

Iceland 27

ideology: a comprehensive set of ideas, often rooted in a particular political philosophy such as liberalism and conservatism, about society and the role of government 39–40

Ikegami, Naoki 52

Immergut, Ellen 35, 38

incremental policy: legislation that brings about small adjustments to the status quo, such as modest expansion of an existing program 37, 38, 39, 49

individual mandate: a law that requires individuals to purchase health insurance, or else pay a fine 16, 35–6, 53, 59, 60

infant mortality rate: the number of children who die under 1 year of age per 1,000 live births 26, 27

Ingram, Helen 46

Institute of Medicine 55

insurance, employment-based 13, 14, 17, 38, 52

insurance, private

    cost containment 13–14

    coverage 3, 11, 12

    lobbying on health reform 34

policies on treatment for depression 23

premiums 12

regulation under ACA 17, 65–6

resistance to foreign lessons 72

interest groups: organized groups whose members share common goals and work toward influencing public policy 34, 36, 40–2, 65

intergovernmental transfers: exchanges of funds between levels of government within a single nation 62

International Obesity Taskforce (IOTF) 26

isolationism: a policy perspective that emphasizes limited international involvement and a focus on domestic ideas and issues 3

Israel 41

Italy 9, 43

J

Jackson, Jeffrey 49

Jacobs, Lawrence 42, 43, 48, 49, 51, 53, 58

Jacobson, Louis 66

James, Chris 48, 49

Japan 8, 22, 27, 52

Jia, H. 25

Jones, Bryan 35

Jones, Jeffrey 55

Jonsson, Egon 51

Jost, Timothy Stoltzfus 65, 66

K

Kaiser Family Foundation 16, 50, 54, 71

Kaiser Health Tracking Poll 36

Katz, Neil 26

Kelley, Ed 56

Kingdon, John 34

Kirkpatrick, David 36

Klein, Ezra 64

Klein, Rudolf 38, 39, 73

Kliff, Sarah 36

Kluckhohn, Clyde 20

Kohut, Andrew 72

Kupat Cholim Clalit (KHC) 41

Kutch, Jessica 1

L

LA Times 39

Land, Gary 4

Lawder, David 1

Le Grand, Julian 9–10, 51, 53

learning lessons from abroad 69–74

Lee, Sang-Yi 9

legislation, health care 13–16 *see also* Patient Protection and Affordable Care Act (ACA)

Lie, Marit 30, 31

life expectancy: the number of years an individual in a particular society is expected to live based on a statistical projection 26, 27

Light, Paul 44

Limbaugh, Rush 1

Lipset, Seymour 3, 25

Liptak, Adam 60

lobbying: the act of attempting to influence public officials and public policy typically in the legislative process 34, 36, 65

Longest, Beaufort 33

longevity analyses 3

Lubetkin, El 25

Lubove, Roy 4

Luke, Douglas 25

Lundgren, Bernt 29

Luxembourg 27, 51

M

MacFarlan, Maitland 50

MacGillis, Alec 37

MacLeod, G.K. 43

managed care: a health care payment and delivery system designed to lower costs by controlling the type, level, and cost of services provided 14

Marmor, Theodore 3, 4, 14, 15, 51, 52

Marmot, Michael 28, 30

Marsh, David 70

Mashaw, Jerry 51, 52

Massachusetts 15–16, 36, 65

Mathews, Anna Wilde 65

McDonough, John 16

McPake, Barbara 73

Mechanic, David 10, 20, 21, 64, 70

Medicaid: a U.S. government health insurance program for low-income individuals and families, funded jointly by the states and federal government 15, 17, 55, 62

Medicare: a U.S. government health insurance program for individuals aged 65 and older, funded primarily through federal payroll taxes 14–15, 54–5

changes under ACA 16, 17, 18, 36

comparative study with British National Health Service 42–3

cost reduction plans 43–4

medicine and culture 20–1

Mertens, Maggie 18

Mexico 50

Modigliani, Andre 34

monopsony: an economic market in which buyers, not suppliers, dominate 51–2

Moore, Michael 4, 71

Moran, Michael 9

morbidity: the proportion of sickness or disease in a specific geographic location, age group, or other segment of society 24

Morone, James 4, 55, 72

Mossialos, Elias 51

Murray, Margaret 49

N

Nathanson, Constance 41

national health expenditures: total annual spending for U.S. health services, including payments for hospital care, physician services, nursing home care, pharmaceuticals, and other types of expenses, by private and public sources 12, 25, 50–1

national health insurance: a universal health insurance system that is financed and administered by a national governing body 4, 8

abroad 22, 38, 40, 41, 52–3

national health systems, classification of 7–10

National Institute for Health and Clinical Excellence (NICE) 24, 64

neocorporatism: a model of cooperative decision-making between government and established interest groups, including employers' organizations and labor unions 42

Netherlands 22, 42, 53

New England Journal of Medicine 55

The New Republic 63

New York Times xi, 10, 36, 38, 71

New Zealand 22, 43

Nielsen Company 25

No Labels movement 39

Norway 29–30, 31, 51

O

Obama, Barack
 reflections on ACA 16, 44–5
 televised address before Congress 10–13
OBAMACARE Repeal Pledge 59
Oberlander, Jonathan 14
obesity: an excessive accumulation of body fat associated with increased health risks, commonly defined by applying a body mass index or some other calculation of ideal body weight 3, 24–6
Ogden, Cynthia 25
Okma, Kieke 3, 4, 41, 42
Organiaation for Economic Co-operation and Development (OECD) 8–9, 12, 25, 48, 50, 51, 54, 56, 66, 67
Orszag, Peter 18
overweight: the state of being above a normal body weight 25
Oxley, Howard 50, 52, 53

P

Palin, Sarah 26, 63
parliamentary systems: a democratic system of government in which the executive branch is directly accountable to the legislature, as opposed to a presidential system which separates these branches 35
Patashnik, Eric 40
Patel, Kant 14
Patient Protection and Affordable Care Act (ACA) 2010 xii, 16–18, 19, 24, 31
 cost-sharing provisions 54–5
 encouragement of competition 53–4
 federal and state responsibilities under 19, 60, 62
 funding of 17–18, 55
 implementation issues 58–60
 individual mandate provision 16, 35–6, 59, 60
 insurance regulation 17, 65–6
 limitations of reform under 18–19, 38, 50
 Obama's reflections on 16, 44–5
 Obama's televised address to Congress 10–13
 policy formulation stage 35–7
 policy tools 47
 quality improvements 55–6
 and rationing 63–5

Payer, Lynne 21

Pear, Robert 17, 24, 38, 65

Perrin, Benjamin 62

Peters, Guy 13, 42

Peterson, Mark 37

pharmaceutical industry 15, 18, 23–4, 36

Picket, Kate 29, 31

placebos: a pseudo medical intervention often given as a control treatment in medical research, such as a pill containing no active agent 24

pluralism: a political philosophy that embraces conflict and compromise among diverse interests as an accepted part of the political process 49

Polder model *see* **neocorporatism**

policy abroad, health

    classifications of national health systems 7–10

    comparative analyses of U.S. and 2–6

    comparative perspective on federalism and 60–3

    interventions 29–31

    learning from 69–74

policy design, health 46–57

    buying power 51–2

    competition and regulation 52–4

    dominant options for 47–50

    and quality issues 55–6

    rising costs 50–1

    tools for 46–7

policy formulation: phase of the policy process during which issues gain a place on the government agenda and legislative solutions are developed and adopted 33, 35–7

policy implementation: phase of the policy process during which laws and programs are put into effect 33, 58–60, 67

policy modification: phase of the policy process that involves the assessment and possible correction or replacement of policies already in existence 33, 35

policy transfer: the process by which knowledge about public policies, administrative arrangements, or institutions is transmitted across time or space 69, 70–1, 72-3

policy venues: institutional structures in which policy decisions get made, e.g., federal or state governments, legislatures, courts, and bureaucracies 35

political culture: citizen attitudes and beliefs that assign meaning to the political process and relate to forms of political behavior 21–2

populist: someone who supports the political interests of ordinary people 26

Portugal 9, 44

Potter, Wendell 72
poverty 17, 28–9
pre-existing conditions: health problems that existed prior to one's application for a
    health insurance policy 16, 17, 36
Preston, Samuel 3
primary care: a patient's principal point of access to the health care system, such as
    a general practitioner, and typically includes the provision of a broad spectrum of
    continuous care and the coordination of additional health services 17, 24
privatization: the transfer of ownership or control of a program or policy activity
    from the public to private sector 15, 69
problem solving, politics of 39–40
psychotherapy: personal counseling with a trained therapist for the treatment of
    psychological problems 24
public opinion: a collection of individual views and attitudes about a particular
    topic, often aggregated for the purpose of consideration in regard to policy issues
    or the performance of government 33, 42–3, 66, 67
    and belief in US health care 1–2, 3–4
"public option" 18, 37
public participation in health care planning 66–7
Puska, Pekka 30
Pye, Lucien 21

Q
Quah, Stella 20
quality of health care see **health care quality**
Quincy, Lynn 55

R
Ramlet, Michael 18
Rapoport, John 51
rationing: the controlled distribution of resources 37, 63–5
Reagan, Michael 10, 15
redistributive taxes: revenues collected by government with the aim of transferring
    resources from wealthier segments of the population to those with lower incomes
    31
reform *see* **health care reform**
regulations: government rules used to guide procedure or behavior that are issued
    by bureaucratic agencies as a new law moves into the implementation phase 58
    on advertising of prescription drugs 23–4
    competition and 52–4
    insurance 17, 65–6

small-area analysis: a study of variations in health care utilization from one community, or small population group, to another 55

social determinants of health: conditions in which one is born, lives, and works that influence health; important factors include economic circumstances, social conditions, discrimination based on factors such as race, ethnicity, gender, or sexual orientation, and the accessibility of health services 26–8

policy interventions abroad 29–31

social insurance: a form of government-supervised coverage in which payroll-based contributions are collected from employers, employees, or both while government makes payments on behalf of those without means 8, 48, 49–50, 64

socialism: an ideology that favors social and economic equality; in socialist societies the means of economic production and distribution are owned and controlled collectively or by a centralized government 14

socialized medicine: a health system that includes public financing and administration of medical services for all; also a term often used pejoratively in the U.S. to characterize reform plans that feature a prominent government role 37, 48

Sommers, Benjamin 62

Soroka, Stuart 48

South Korea 8

Soviet Union 8

Spain 9, 44, 54

The Spirit Level 29

Ståhl, Timo 30

State Children's Health Insurance Program: a U.S. government health program that provides federal matching dollars to states that provide health insurance to low-income children who are not eligible for Medicaid 15

states' role in health care system 15–16

and challenges of ACA 19, 60, 62

Stokes, Bruce 72

Stolberg, Sheryl 10, 38

Stone, Deborah 4, 31, 34

Stone, Diane 69, 70

Stone, Peter 36

Stremikis, Kristof 2

studies of health care, comparative international 2–6

Sweden 22, 27, 29

Switzerland 53, 54

Szabo, Liz 23

T

Taiwan 8–9

Tantaros, Andrea 64

taxation 17–18, 31, 48, 53

Tenth Amendment: part of the U.S. Constitution's Bill of Rights, guaranteeing that all powers not granted to the federal government or prohibited to the states are reserved to the states 60

Thatcher, Margaret 38–9, 53

Thomma, Steven 31

Truman, Benedict 31

Tuohy, Carolyn 48

Twaddle, Andrew 41

typology: a systematic classification of types or categories 9–10

U

underinsured: individuals who have health insurance coverage that is inadequate because it fails to cover needed services and/or exposes the individual to costs that amount to a substantial portion of personal income 11

uninsured: individuals not covered by health insurance 11, 13, 18

program for children 15

unitary political systems: systems of government with one central authority and localities possess limited autonomy 60

United Kingdom

anti-obesity policies 26

comparative study of Medicare with National Health Service 42–3

evidence-based medicine promoted in 64

health policy 4, 38–9, 52–3, 54

political culture 22

universality: a scenario in which 100 percent of a society's population has health care coverage 11, 49, 50

U.S. Census Bureau 11, 13, 14

V

Vasoodaven, Vilashiny 53

veto: exercise of a power held by the U.S. president to block legislation from becoming law by withholding his signature; overcoming a presidential veto requires a two-thirds vote in Congress 59

veto points: opportunities in which lawmakers find they have the ability to block legislation from moving forward; for official veto power, see **veto** 35, 38

Visscher, Tommy 24

W

Wall Street Journal 12, 63, 65

Wasem, Jürgen 66
Weaver, Christopher 65
Weil, Alan 60, 62
Weisman, Jonathan 12
Weissert, Carol and William 34
Whitaker, Robert 23
White, Joseph 4
Whitehead, Margaret 27, 28, 29
Whitman, Glen 3
Wilkinson, Richard 29, 31
Wilsford, David 38
Wonca 24
World Health Organization 2, 23, 24, 26, 27, 28, 30, 38, 44
Wörz, Markus 52

X
xenophobia: a fear or dislike of strangers or foreigners 6

Z
Zaharoff, Josh 36
Zeleny, Jeff 10, 39
Zimbabwe 27